D0516996

The Premature Baby Book

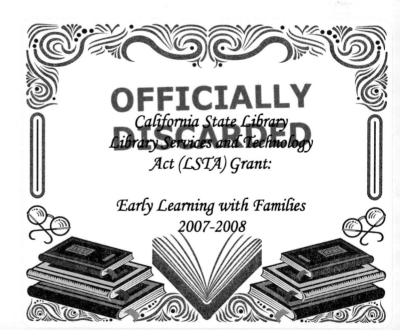

OFFICIALLY DISCARDED

California State Library
Library Services and Technology
Act (LSTA) Grant:

Early Learning with Families
2007-2008

Sears Parenting Library

The Pregnancy Book

The Baby Book

The Birth Book

The Attachment Parenting Book

The Breastfeeding Book

The Fussy Baby Book

The Discipline Book

The Family Nutrition Book

The A.D.D. Book

The Successful Child

Parenting.com FAQ Books

The First Three Months

How to Get Your Baby to Sleep

Keeping Your Baby Healthy

Feeding the Picky Eater

Sears Children's Library

Baby on the Way

What Baby Needs

Eat Healthy, Feel Great

You Can Go to the Potty

The Premature Baby Book

Everything You Need to Know About Your Premature Baby
From Birth to Age One

WILLIAM SEARS, M.D. , ROBERT SEARS, M.D.,
JAMES SEARS, M.D. , AND MARTHA SEARS, R.N.

LITTLE, BROWN AND COMPANY
New York ◆ Boston ◆ London

Little, Brown and Company
Hachette Book Group USA
237 Park Avenue, New York, NY 10017

Visit our Web site at www.HachetteBookGroupUSA.com

FIRST EDITION

Stethoscope image courtesy of New Vision Technologies Inc.

Library of Congress Cataloging-in-Publication Data

The premature baby book : everything you need to know about your premature baby from birth to age one / William Sears . . . [et al.]. — 1st ed.
      p.   cm. — (Sears parenting library)
    Includes index.
    ISBN 978-0-316-73822-4
    1. Infants (Premature).   2. Infants (Premature) — Care.
3. Parent and infant.   4. Parent and child.   I. Sears, William, M.D.

RJ250.P723   2004
618.92'011 — dc22   2004001414

10   9   8   7   6   5   4   3   2

Q-FF

Designed by Jeanne Abboud
Drawings by Deborah Maze

PRINTED IN THE UNITED STATES OF AMERICA

Contents

VISIT DR. SEARS ONLINE

www.AskDrSears.com

Now you can access thousands of pages of pediatric medical and parenting information. Our comprehensive online resource, personally written by the Doctors Sears, expands on many of the topics discussed in *The Premature Baby Book*. We continuously update the health information on our website to provide you with the latest in parenting and health care issues. AskDrSears.com offers valuable insights on such topics as Pregnancy and Childbirth, Infant Feeding, Family Nutrition, Discipline and Behavior, Fussy Babies, and Sleep Problems.

Our website also includes these unique features:

- Dr. Sears's Medicine Cabinet, a comprehensive guide to over-the-counter medications, including specific dose information
- Childhood Illnesses, detailed medical information on many common, and not-so-common, child and family illnesses
- Monthly Pediatric Health News Updates
- Seasonal Pediatric Health Alerts
- Valuable month-by-month parenting and medical advice to complement your child's regular checkups
- Frequently Asked Questions answered
- Personal words of encouragement and humor from the daily lives of the Doctors Sears
- *The Premature Baby Book* updates. We will post any significant changes to *The Premature Baby Book* (and all our books) to provide you with the most accurate and up-to-date medical information.

A Word from Dr. Bill

Early in my pediatric career I had the privilege of being a "preemie doctor." After spending five months as a resident in the Neonatal Intensive Care Unit of the Hospital for Sick Children in Toronto, the largest children's hospital in the world, I went on to become an associate ward chief in this NICU, a position I held for the next four years. In the mornings, I would supervise and teach pediatric interns and residents in the NICU, and in the afternoon, I would see many of the NICU "graduates" in my office for routine pediatric care. I enjoyed the best of both worlds as a pediatrician: the medical challenges of the high-tech NICU, and the fun of watching babies grow up in a general pediatric practice.

An exciting change from when I worked in the NICU in the 1970s is the amazing survival of younger and smaller preemies today. I remember we used to give a 3-pound preemie only a 50 percent chance of survival, and a 1- or 2-pound preemie had an even grimmer prognosis. Now I am excited to see virtually all "3-pounders" thrive, most without any long-term complications, and more than half of

1-pound preemies survive. Modern neonatology care is nothing short of miraculous.

While it has been many years since I was the doctor in charge of hospitalized preemies, I have continued to care for NICU graduates in my office. Working together, my sons, Dr. Jim and Dr. Bob, who are now my partners in the Sears Family Pediatric Practice, my wife, Martha, who as a lactation consultant has helped many mothers work through the challenges of breastfeeding a preemie, and I have learned what helps parents of preemies and their babies thrive. Not only do we enjoy watching the babies grow, but we also find it very rewarding to watch the parents grow to become capable, sensitive caregivers.

After years of observing babies and parents together, we have come to believe that the need level phenomenon is at work in special ways in parents of preemies. Every baby is born with certain needs. Some babies, especially preemies, have greater and more complex needs than other babies have. Premature infants needed more time in the womb but didn't get it. So they need more care outside the womb to make up for lost time. When parents are given accurate information and are empowered with parenting tools that nurture their attachment to their baby, their caregiving skills rise to a higher level, a level that matches the higher need level of their preemie. As a result, parents and their preemies bring out the best in one another.

Throughout the first few weeks or even months of your preemie's life, you may feel overwhelmed by the high-tech medical care. All the machines and medicines will help make it possible for you to take a healthy baby home from the hospital, but they may leave you feeling like an outsider, not a parent. For your own sake and that of your baby, you need to get involved in your preemie's care. Yet there will be times when you don't want to be "part of the medical team" or to become a wizard in medical technology. You just want to be the best mother or father you can be for your baby. While the medical team can take care of baby's physical needs, it's up to you to make it possible for your baby to thrive. "Thriving" means not only growing by getting heavier and taller, it means growing physically, intellectually, and emotionally.

When we were interviewing parents of preemies about what they felt a book on caring for their baby should contain, we frequently heard, "I'm tired of books telling me everything that can go wrong!" Instead, we have taken a positive approach. *The Premature Baby Book* focuses on what parents can do to lessen the chances of things going wrong. Throughout the book you will find helpful tips, shared feelings, and lessons learned from parents who have been there before you. Their words appear in short italicized sections.

Because of advances in neonatal care, nowadays most preemies survive and grow. Yet, whether or not your baby thrives depends not only on the medical care but also on the special care you provide. What helps babies thrive? Interaction with other human beings. You nurture your baby with your milk, your eyes, your voice, your skin, your touch, your love. Others may have the special knowledge to help your baby overcome medical challenges, but you are the person most dedicated to giving your special baby a special kind of parenting. Let's get started!

1

Parenting Your Preemie in the Hospital

Welcome to the world of the Neonatal Intensive Care Unit. Certainly this is not the environment in which you had envisioned yourself caring for your newborn. Suddenly you are no longer an ordinary mom or an ordinary dad, and you may be feeling overwhelmed by the complexity of your baby's medical care. We have learned that the more parents know about the care their baby is receiving, the better they cope with the stress of having a baby in the NICU. And the better they cope, the better they parent their baby, doing the things that only Mom and Dad can do. In the following chapters, you will learn about life in the NICU: what special care your baby needs, what problems may occur, and, above all, how you can help. In the first chapter, we will address the questions we hear most often from parents of preemies. We will take you on a tour of the NICU, introduce you to some very important persons in your baby's life, and help you learn how best to communicate with them. We will then take you on a head-to-toe, system-by-system tour of your preemie's unique features and needs. With this information, you will be able to participate in your baby's care. Committed parents can meet their baby's needs in ways that busy nurses cannot. Finally, we will help you work through the fears and feelings that most parents of preemies experience. We will also learn from the "experts," parents of preemies who have shared helpful caregiving tips and lessons they have learned. Our goal in the first part of this book is to help you become a keen observer of your preemie's unique needs and empower you to meet them.

The First Day — The Top 10 Questions About Premature Babies

DURING PREGNANCY, parents dream of those magical moments after birth when they will meet their new baby: those first moments of bonding, of gazing deeply, with wonder, into their newborn's questioning eyes. They look forward to skin-to-skin contact, to baby's first suckling at the breast, to holding baby close to their heart. These pre-natal visions of the birth experience are important. They prepare you to love your baby.

Parents of a baby born prematurely do not get to experience the fulfillment of these dreams right away. They are challenged with a different beginning to their baby's life. Instead of holding and comforting their new bundle of joy in their arms, they find their arms empty. Instead of reading helpful handouts from the nurses about caring for their newborn, they must scrutinize the fine print on a consent form that authorizes any and all necessary treatments their baby may need in the Neonatal Intensive Care Unit, or, as you will come to know it, the NICU. Instead of learning to recognize and respond to their own baby's unique cry, they must

endure the cries of healthy newborns in the hospital hallway. When Mom and Dad look at each other, they don't see joy and excitement. They see only worry.

Not all parents of premature babies go through such an abrupt and dramatic break from the expected newborn routine. Every baby's start in life is different. Some premature babies are born with mature lungs, and their condition is very stable right from the start. These babies and their parents may enjoy several hours together before the baby is taken to the hospital nursery. Other babies are accompanied to the NICU by the father or a friend or family member, who will learn right away that the baby is doing well, despite the need for special care. Other babies are born with very immature lungs and struggle right from birth. For these families, the delivery room is a place of drama and uncertainty. Their baby is immediately whisked away to the NICU, where he or she is surrounded by doctors, nurses, flashing lights, beeping monitors, tubes, and sensors.

What do parents feel in those first hours? Worry. Fear. Loss. These are natural reactions that anyone would experience in this situation. But perhaps the most pervasive feeling at this early stage is *uncertainty*. You wonder, Where is my baby? How is my baby doing? Is my baby fighting for his little life? What do the doctors and nurses think? Is my baby worse off than I fear, or not so bad? This initial period of not knowing exactly how your baby is doing can be tough, especially if you are not able to be with your premature newborn during the first few hours in the NICU. A hundred questions go through your mind, and there are few immediate answers.

Whether you begin reading this book in the first hours after birth, when you are still very uncertain about what lies ahead for your baby, or later, when your baby's condition is stable and you know more about what to expect, there are probably many things you wish to know. We have written this chapter to answer the questions most parents ask in the first hours and days after their baby's premature birth. We have relied on "experts" — parents of preemies — to tell us what mothers and fathers most want to know at this stage. (You will find comments from these parents throughout the book.)

1. How premature is my baby, and will my baby be okay?

When your baby is born prematurely, your immediate concern is whether or not he will be all right. How serious is the situation when baby is born at 34 weeks' gestation? At 28 weeks' gestation? Will your baby have any long-term medical or developmental problems? How likely is it that your baby will have a "normal," healthy life? Unfortunately, the answers

you want most are the ones your doctors are not able to give — at least not yet. They must first assess your baby's condition and see how he responds to initial supportive measures.

In general, the earlier a baby is born, the more likely she may be to have short-term or long-term difficulties. The baby's weight at birth also affects the outcome. However, every baby is unique, and every baby responds differently to the challenges of coming into this world early. It is entirely possible that a baby born at 34 weeks will have a more difficult course than a baby born at 29 weeks.

Dr. Bob notes: Recently, I had the pleasure of doing a checkup on a beautiful five-year-old girl named Maria, who was a new patient. After giving her a clean bill of health and finding no developmental or learning problems, I asked her mother if Maria had experienced any major medical problems in the past. I was surprised when she told me that her child had been born at 28 weeks' gestation. Despite being born almost 3 months early, she had encountered no long-term health problems whatsoever.

This child is just one example of how the dramatic advances in neonatology are helping more premature babies not only survive but also live normal, healthy lives. While some babies will have ongoing medical or developmental challenges once they leave the NICU, the majority of preemies grow up just fine.

2. What caused my baby to be born prematurely?

The first question anybody asks when hardship comes along is why? It is natural for parents to ask themselves, "Why did this happen?" "What did I do to cause this?" "What could I have done to prevent this?"

There are a number of medical conditions during pregnancy that can lead to premature birth (we will discuss these shortly), but in most cases, premature birth comes without warning and has no apparent medical cause. A mother who has a normal pregnancy with no detectable medical conditions and who receives regular prenatal care may still give birth prematurely. There is absolutely nothing she did to cause her baby to be born prematurely, and there is nothing she could have done to prevent the premature birth. Even if a woman has a complication during her pregnancy that leads to a prematurely born baby, such a complication also happens by chance, and again, there is nothing she did to cause it. For example, a woman may develop preeclampsia (high blood pressure) during her pregnancy, and this may induce premature labor, but usually there is nothing she could have done to prevent the preeclampsia. This is true for all of the causes of premature birth discussed below.

Known medical conditions that make a premature birth more likely include the following:

- previous premature birth, miscarriage, or multiple abortions
- history of kidney disease
- structural problems in the uterus: a weakened cervix, heart-shaped uterus, or bifid uterus (uterus divided into two separate parts)
- prenatal complications: placental problems, too much or too little amniotic fluid, uterine fibroids (benign growths), preeclampsia or toxemia, early rupture

of the membranes (your water breaks too early), or infection of the uterus
- multiple babies: twins, triplets, or more have a greater chance of being born prematurely
- obesity
- being very underweight from undernourishment

Three factors that can increase the risk of prematurity *are* under a woman's control:

- *Cigarette smoking* retards the growth of the placenta and can therefore lead to an early birth.

A NOTE FOR DADS

This is a very emotional time for both you and your wife. Even though your baby's early entry into the world is *not* your wife's fault, she may believe in her heart that she could have prevented it. It is crucial to be supportive and sensitive to her as she deals with her unfounded guilt. If she feels that you blame her for your baby's premature birth, this can create a huge strain on your relationship at a time when you need to be strong together. Get the facts about the situation, resolve your own feelings, and move ahead.

Dads are often the first to get their hands on the baby while Mother is recovering, oftentimes from a cesarean. Mother then feels isolated and waits for a report from Dad. Be sure you update your wife on your baby's condition as often as you can. Don't keep her worrying in the dark.

PREEMIE STATS

More than 450,000 babies are born prematurely each year in the United States, about 12 percent of all births. Newborns are grouped into the following categories, according to their birth weight and gestation:

- *Full-term baby.* Any baby born at 37 weeks' gestation or later is not considered premature. A full-term baby typically weighs more than 5½ pounds (2500 grams)
- *Mildly premature (35 to 36 weeks).* These babies usually weigh between 3½ and 7 pounds (1600 to 3200 grams), and, since they are only 3 to 5 weeks early, they have a survival rate of 98 to 100 percent. They typically have no immediate breathing problems or long-term complications, and they often do not even need to go to the NICU.
- *Moderately premature (30 to 34 weeks).* These babies typically weigh between 2½ and 5½ pounds (1100 to 2500 grams) and have a survival rate slightly greater than 98 percent. Babies born at this age and size often have immature lungs and require some assistance in breathing at first. The younger the infant and the lower the birth weight, the more likely it is that a baby will need special assistance in the NICU. Most of these babies will have no long-term medical issues.
- *Extremely premature (26 to 29 weeks).* Babies born this early weigh between 1½ and 3½ pounds (750 to 1600 grams). The survival rate for the earliest and smallest in this group is around 90 percent. Nearly all extremely premature babies have immature lungs and require breathing assistance from a ventilator for a period of time. Even though survival rates in this group are excellent, the risk of long-term problems is higher, although one recent research study showed some very encouraging sta-

- *Drug abuse* can lead to many pregnancy complications, including premature birth.
- *Lack of adequate prenatal care* increases the risk of prematurity. When prenatal complications are identified and treated early, a premature birth may be prevented.

Aside from these last three factors, there is nothing a woman does to cause, and nothing she can do to prevent, the premature birth of her baby. It is important to resolve any feelings of guilt or blame you may have and move on to focusing on

your baby. If you need to know more about why your baby was born early, talk with your birth attendant. Or ask your nurse if you can speak with a hospital chaplain or counselor to help you address these feelings.

3. What is happening to my baby right now?

The frustrating, helpless feelings you may have on your baby's first day may come from not knowing what your baby is going through. You may wonder, How is my tistics. Among infants with birth weights greater than 1000 grams (2½ pounds), 95 percent not only survived but had no severe long-term health problems.

- *Micropreemies (less than 26 weeks).* These babies weigh less than 1¾ pounds (750 grams). This group once had an almost 100 percent fatality rate, but with recent advances in neonatal care, 25 to 50 percent of these babies now survive. Over half of micropreemies will have a number of long-term problems, such as visual and neurologic deficits and chronic lung problems.
- Some NICUs classify preemies based on weight alone. *Low birth weight babies* (LBW — weight between 1500 and 2500 grams, or 3½ to 5½ pounds); *very low birth weight babies* (VLBW — weight less than 1600 grams, or 3½ pounds); and *extremely low birth weight babies* (ELBW — weight less than 750 grams, or 1¾ pounds). These weight groupings are often used in

research studies of premature babies.

As you can see, each extra week in the womb increases baby's chances of growing up healthy and strong. If your baby is only mildly to moderately premature, she has an outstanding chance of survival and will most likely not have any long-term challenges. If your baby has been born extremely premature, or is classified as a micropreemie, then you and your baby may face many challenges in the coming weeks and in the years ahead.

Remember, statistics are just numbers. Your baby is an individual. Also, keep in mind that many of the "poor outcome" statistics you may encounter in books or on Internet sites are old and do not reflect the newest advances in neonatal (and parental) care. In the pages to come, we will share with you many ideas you can use to improve your baby's chances of surviving and thriving.

baby doing? What exactly is being done for my baby right now? Why does my baby need so many wires and tubes? What does all that equipment and monitoring actually do? Is my baby in pain? In the next chapter, we will explain in detail the medical procedures and equipment that are used to care for your baby. For now, here's a brief discussion of what typically happens to a premature baby during the first twenty-four hours. This basic understanding of what's happening may be all you need at this stage. As your baby's condition stabilizes and you spend more

time at her side, you can learn more details about your baby's care. If you are reading this book when your baby is already a few weeks old, then the following information may give you some insight into what happened during that hectic first day.

Doctors' first concern in the hours after baby's birth is his respiratory status. How well are his lungs working? Are the lungs mature enough to provide oxygen to the body unassisted? Over the first twenty-four to forty-eight hours, the doctors and nurses will closely monitor baby's respiratory

---

UNDERSTANDING HELPS COPING

The more you understand all the procedures involved in the special care of your preemie, the better you are able to cope and the more you can help.

---

status and observe his breathing pattern carefully. Is he breathing comfortably, or is his breathing becoming more rapid, shallow, and strained?

The level of oxygen in his blood is monitored using a sensor taped to his hand or foot, as well as with blood tests.

At this point, premature babies fall into one of two categories: those whose lungs are mature enough to handle the transition from the womb into open air, and those who temporarily need assistance with breathing.

Babies with mature lungs may need nothing more than some oxygen blown into their nose to make breathing a bit easier. Many infants, however, especially those born before 32 weeks, have immature lungs that are not ready to absorb oxygen correctly. This may be immediately apparent in the delivery room, or the doctors and nurses may conclude after several hours of observation that baby's breathing is becoming more labored. If your baby is not breathing adequately on his own, a breathing tube is inserted through his mouth into his lungs. This procedure is called intubation. The tube is attached to a machine called a ventilator, which breathes for your baby. As baby's lungs start to mature and absorb oxygen better, his reliance on the ventilator will decrease. Depending on the degree of prematurity, babies can require ventilation

for as little as a few hours or as long as several weeks. If your baby needs intensive respiratory support, do not worry that he is stressed or in pain. Babies are given relaxing and pain-relieving medications during this invasive period. They generally sleep through most of it.

An intravenous line (an IV) will be placed in your baby's umbilical cord. This site provides easy access to blood samples for testing. Baby will also receive fluids through the IV, since he won't be able to eat right away.

*Don't drown yourself in information. The Internet is a wonderful thing, but it can make you crazy. Your child is unique and so is your situation. There is no way you can predict the outcome by reading about all the possibilities.**

4. *Why is my baby being transferred to another hospital?*

If your baby is born in a large hospital with a busy obstetrics unit, chances are that the neonatal nursery there is equipped to care for your premature baby. However, if your baby is born at a small suburban or rural hospital, your baby may need to be transferred to a larger hospital with a higher-level nursery. Neonatal nurseries are classified by their ability to handle complex problems:

Basic Care Nursery (formerly called Level I). Any hospital that has an obstetrics unit has at least a Basic Care Nursery. It is equipped to handle healthy babies

---

* Throughout this book, you will hear from the experts —
moms and dads who share their feelings and offer tips
about being the parent of a preemie.

born at 35 weeks' gestation or older who do not have any respiratory or other significant medical problems. This type of unit has a pediatrician (or sometimes a neonatologist) available to handle unexpected complications and stabilize a sick baby for transport to a larger hospital. If your baby is born prior to 35 weeks, weighs less than 4 pounds (1800 grams), or has any significant breathing problems regardless of gestational age, she will probably be transferred to a Specialty Care NICU (see below).

Specialty Care NICU (formerly Level II). Found in many large urban hospitals and most large rural regional medical centers, this type of NICU is well equipped and staffed by full-time neonatologists. A Specialty Care Unit is able to care for most premature babies born at 32 weeks or later and can care for babies with moderate but stable problems that are expected to improve quickly.

Subspecialty Care NICU (formerly Level III). This more advanced type of unit is usually found in most major university hospitals and large medical centers. It cares for premature babies with moderate to severe complications, including birth defects, that require specialized care from pediatric subspecialists, such as surgeons, cardiologists, neurologists, neurosurgeons, and radiologists.

5. How can I help care for my baby in the NICU?

Every parent's natural impulse is to help their child who is hurt or sick. But when a premature baby goes to the NICU, many parents feel helpless. You want to do something for your sick baby, but there seems to be nothing you can do. You may try to shut down this impulse to help and settle for feeling helpless, or your helping energy may get diverted into worrying or trying to control things over which you have little influence.

Take heart! There actually are many things you can do to help your baby, both immediately and throughout the NICU stay. Your involvement with your baby at this time is critical, for both of you. Here are several ways you can help your baby:

Provide breast milk. A mother of a premature baby may decide that she might as well resign herself to the fact that she won't be able to breastfeed. Or the parents of a preemie may feel that breastfeeding is bound to fail, since the normal pattern for the beginning of the feeding process has been disrupted. Nothing is further from the truth. Not only will you eventually be able to breastfeed your baby, but it is critical for your baby's health that he receive breast milk as soon as feeding is possible. Giving your milk to your baby is so important that we devote two chapters to this subject. In chapters 6 and 7 we will discuss in detail how you can provide breast milk and eventually breastfeed your baby, as well as explain the numerous medical benefits of giving your baby breast milk, but here's what you need to know right away.

As soon as you feel ready, ask the nurse about pumping your breasts. The sooner you start, the better. Pump every three hours or as often as possible. Use a hospital-grade electric breast pump with a double pumping kit, so that you can pump both breasts at the same time. Ask to have a breast pump in your hospital room and begin storing all the milk you pump. You will start off getting very little, but every little bit adds up. This is probably the single most important thing you can do for your baby. Some preemies can be fed breast milk in the first day of life, depending on a variety of factors.

If the thought of breastfeeding overwhelms you right now, and you are worried that it might be too stressful for you and baby, realize that actual breastfeeding may be several weeks away. You will be much more able to face these challenges at that time. In the meanwhile, pumping your milk will give your baby the best nutrition possible.

If I felt he was too warm or too cold, they would let me fix it.

Get attached to your baby. The quiet, focused time that a mother, father, and baby spend together in the hours and days after birth helps the parent-infant relationship get off to a good start. When parents are separated from their baby after birth because of medical problems, the usual bonding process is disrupted. Finding opportunities to get attached to their baby is vital to the emotional well-being of both parents. One way to do this is to begin spending time in the nursery, touching your premature baby. If your baby is relatively stable and needs little intervention, you will be able to hold him right away. If your baby is on a ventilator to assist his breathing, you may not be able to hold him, but you can still touch him, gently kiss him, and speak to him. Spend as much time with your baby as you can, right from the start. Not only will you benefit from this early bonding, but research

has shown that preemies are more stable and grow better when they spend more time physically in touch with their parents.

Begin "kangaroo care." This type of parent involvement in the care of a premature newborn is modeled after the way a kangaroo cares for its young. A baby kangaroo is born at a very early stage of development — like a premature baby — and spends many weeks living inside the mom's pouch, where it is nourished and kept warm. Kangaroo care for your baby involves holding your baby skin-to-skin for many hours each day. In chapter 5 we will provide a crash course in how to do K care as well as discuss the research that has shown how K care can greatly benefit a premature baby.

Dr. Jim advises: Years down the road, you want to have no regrets. Don't let fears about the future and the problems your preemie may develop keep you from expressing your love and concern for him through touch, soft words, and time spent together. Whatever happens in the days to come, you will know that you gave him your best. Take full advantage of every moment.

Become involved. Mom and Dad are both a valuable part of the medical team. It is easy to let yourselves be overwhelmed by all the high-tech equipment that you see around your baby in the NICU and by the medical terminology used by the staff. While there are many things that you cannot do for your baby in the NICU, your level of involvement and daily interest in your baby's care will be noticed by the

NICU staff. The more they see of you, the more they will respect and seek your input in decisions made about your baby's care.

6. When will I be able to hold and breastfeed my baby?

Usually, parents are allowed to hold their baby as soon as he is off the ventilator. For extremely premature babies, this will be several weeks after birth. You can certainly touch and caress your baby during this time. If your baby does not require a ventilator, you should be able to hold him right away.

A baby's age and medical situation play a significant role in determining when he will be able to breastfeed. Babies generally do not develop the physical ability to suck and swallow efficiently, either with a bottle or at the breast, until around 32 to 34 weeks of age. Prior to that time, babies are fed pumped human milk or infant formula through a tube that goes down their nose or mouth into the stomach. Once a baby is mature enough to suck properly and stable enough to be put to the breast, it is time to begin breastfeeding. Some babies may continue to have minor breathing difficulties for several days after they come off the ventilator, and this may delay breastfeeding until the breathing stabilizes. See chapters 5 and 6 for more detailed breastfeeding information.

7. How long will my baby have to stay in the hospital?

There is no magic age or target weight at which every baby gets to go home from the NICU. A general rule is that you will be able to take your baby home by his expected date of birth. Many babies go home sooner than this if they do not encounter any major setbacks. Often a baby does so well that she is ready to go home weeks before the medical team anticipated. Sometimes minor problems arise that delay a baby's discharge for several days or more. If your baby is born extremely premature, you can expect her to spend several months in the NICU. If she is only moderately premature and doesn't require a ventilator for assistance in breathing, you may be able to take her home within several weeks.

Keep your hopes high, but without a timetable.

8. Will my medical insurance pay for my baby's care in the NICU?

Almost all standard PPO and HMO insurance plans will cover the cost of your baby's care in the NICU. Call your insurance company as soon as you can (preferably within the first day or two) to make sure your baby is enrolled in your plan and to ask about coverage. Find out right away whether you have the option to modify your plan to a small deductible or none at all, since you can expect to reach the limit on the deductible amount while your baby is hospitalized. It can also be helpful to meet with the hospital financial advisor to verify your insurance coverage. If you do not have medical insurance, the advisor will be able to guide you toward a financial aid program.

The hospital social worker is another valuable resource. He or she can help you determine which federal assistance programs you may qualify for, and put you in contact with local organizations that offer financial assistance for medical bills and nonmedical costs, such as food and parking, which can really add up over a long NICU stay.

9. Will my baby need special care after leaving the hospital?

The amount of special care your baby may need once you go home depends on a variety of factors. Many preemies graduate from the NICU quickly and go home without needing any special care. Some need frequent weight checks at the pediatrician's office or in the follow-up clinic at the hospital. Some babies go home with a monitor to use when baby is unattended to check on heart rate and breathing during sleep. A few preemies with feeding or breathing problems may require special tube feedings, breathing treatments, or occasional oxygen. Most preemies go home needing only the "special care" of a loving family to help them grow and thrive just like any full-term baby. In chapters 9 and 12, we discuss various medical challenges that your baby may face and the type of special care that may be needed during baby's first years of life.

10. Will my baby develop like a full-term baby?

While every baby develops at his own unique pace, you can expect that your baby will meet developmental milestones based on his gestational age (also called corrected chronological age, or CCA), and not his actual age. For example, a baby who is actually 4 months old but who was born 2 months early has a CCA age of only 2 months. His development is therefore comparable to that of a full-term 2-month-old. Many full-term 2-month-olds begin to laugh and coo at this stage. The baby who was born 2 months early wouldn't be expected to laugh and coo until 4 months after his birthday. Your baby may catch up to his full-term peers around one to two years of age. See chapter 11 for more on infant development.

Dr. Bob advises: Concentrate on becoming knowledgeable about your baby's present situation and her day-to-day progress rather than concerning yourself with long-term developmental issues. Take things one day or, at most, one week at a time. In the days before baby is discharged from the hospital, you may want to ask more questions and become informed about any problems your baby is likely to face. By that time, the doctors will have a more accurate sense of how your baby will fare, and you will be ready to look a little farther into the future. In these early days, try not to clutter your mind with worries about what-ifs that may never come to pass.

You have been blessed and challenged with a baby who was born prematurely but who is, first and foremost, your own special son or daughter. We hope that these introductory questions and answers have given you a better understanding of your baby's situation and that you will use this knowledge immediately to become involved in the care of your newborn. The rest of this book will help you to both understand more about your baby's medical care and feel comfortable in the NICU.

PREPARING FOR A PREEMIE

If you know ahead of time that you are at risk for premature delivery because of a multiple pregnancy or medical complications, you have the opportunity to prepare yourself for the days your baby will spend in the NICU. It's hard to learn the ropes when you are sleep deprived, postpartum, and sad about being separated from your baby. Tour the NICU, if possible, during pregnancy. Familiarize yourself with the NICU environment and available resources *before* you need them.

The NICU quickly became my home away from home.

Rehearse your delivery. Decide beforehand whether your partner will stay with you after delivery or accompany your baby to the NICU. Ask if you can have a brief glimpse of your baby or hold him for a few minutes before he is whisked away. Plan to have a relative or close friend present at the birth who will stay with you immediately postpartum if your partner is going to leave with the baby. You may want someone to talk to or someone who can carry messages from the NICU about your baby's condition.

Acknowledge your feelings. Watching baby be whisked off to the NICU after birth will be hard. People around you — friends, family, medical staff — may tell you to dry your tears and be glad that baby is being well cared for. Don't let them tell you that your feelings of loss don't matter.

Obtain a breast pump. Arrange to have a breast pump in your postpartum hospital room. Find out if the NICU will supply you with a pump to use later at home or if you must arrange to rent one. Learn how to assemble and operate your pump, even prior to delivery. Most insurance companies will cover the rental fees for a pump, although you may need a letter from the doctor, stating that breast milk is medically necessary for your baby. If your health insurance company balks at paying for a breast pump, fight for reimbursement of these expenses. Giving baby your breast milk will save your insurance company a lot of money. If your baby were getting formula in the hospital, the company would pay for that. If your insurance company balks at paying for the pump, keep fighting. After all, your milk is your baby's best preventive medicine.

Consult a lactation specialist. Find out if the hospital or NICU provides lactation consultant services. If not, find a lactation consultant in your community to help you with pumping and breastfeeding problems.

Check your insurance. Find out what medical insurance will cover and what it won't. Out-of-pocket expenses can really add up. Talk to the hospital billing department and your insurance company to get an idea of what you will have to pay. You can then make plans for minimizing your out-of-pocket expenses and paying your share of baby's hospital bill.

2

Navigating the NICU

Our time in the hospital was the most emotionally grueling experience of my life. Forget the Hallmark moments of bringing your newborn baby to your breast, posing for pictures in the recovery room. . . . Welcome instead to the world of intimate bonding sessions with your breast pump at 2 a.m., peeling and chapped hands from hospital antibacterial soap, total strangers spending more time than you with your baby, and the endless beeping of computers monitoring vital signs. This is the life of a NICU mom.

FIRST IMPRESSIONS

Your first visit to the NICU (Neonatal Intensive Care Unit) may be a shock. Rows of baby incubators, flashing monitors, beeping alarms, and tiny babies attached to wires and IV tubes are enough to overwhelm even the bravest heart. You will meet many different kinds of medical personnel, encounter unfamiliar equipment and procedures, and be surrounded by sick babies and worried parents. All of this can be alarming and confusing. But amid the hectic high-tech hustle and bustle,

there is a sense of order. Everybody has a job to do, and everyone does it well.

You are a VIP, a very important person in your baby's care. In this chapter, we will introduce you to life in the NICU. We will tell you about the various medical personnel involved in your baby's care and explain the purpose of the medical equipment that is used to care for your baby. We hope that after reading this chapter, you will feel more comfortable and confident about becoming intimately involved in your baby's care.

First Visit with Your Baby

Which baby is mine? may be the foremost question in your mind as you first enter the NICU. If you are reading this book in preparation for an expected premature birth, or if you are just now preparing for your first visit to your brand-new baby in the NICU, this section will help you understand what you may see on your way to your baby's bedside. If you have already spent some time with your baby in the NICU, this chapter will help you understand the things you have already seen.

When you enter the NICU, you'll find yourself in a world completely foreign. There is a lot to look at. There are rarely any private rooms in a neonatal nursery. Babies share one or several large rooms. If it is a large and busy unit, on the way to see your infant, you may walk past dozens of babies requiring various levels of care. Some babies will be hooked up to multiple monitors, IVs, and breathing machines and will be lying on open treatment platforms or inside incubator cribs. Others may simply be swaddled in a blanket while lying peacefully in a small open bassinet.

Be prepared to be wheeled up to see your baby for the first time only to be handed a bunch of papers and stuff to sign first. That just goes with the territory. Remember, hospitals have to do their job, too, and the paperwork is just a temporary inconvenience.

Stable babies. If your baby was born just a few weeks early, was stable in the delivery room, and is in the NICU mainly for observation, you probably won't find the technology surrounding her too overwhelming. For the first several hours in the NICU, your baby will be placed on an open table under a warming lamp. You may see a sensor for the oxygen monitor taped to her foot, and perhaps the wire for the heart rate monitor taped to her chest. Your baby may be wearing only a diaper. This makes it easier for the NICU nurse, who is probably hovering nearby, to assess her breathing pattern, color, and body temperature. The heat lamp will keep your baby warm.

Check with the nurse to be sure, but you can probably touch your baby (with well-washed hands, of course), explore her little body, stroke her head and tummy, and massage her hands and feet. Don't think of the NICU as a hands-off place, though a preemie may appear fragile. These early visits are a perfect opportunity for you to begin to get to know and love your baby. Ask for a chair so you can sit by your baby, and ask if you can hold her. Holding her won't interfere with baby's simple heart and oxygen monitors. This early hands-on session does good things for both baby and parents. Research has shown that a caregiver's touch helps regulate baby's breathing and heart rate. And being close to your baby will bring out your parenting instincts and help you realize your little preemie isn't so fragile after all. Early physical contact also does good things for breastfeeding mothers. This closeness stimulates the mothering hormone prolactin and increases breast milk production.

If several hours have passed since the birth and your baby's breathing and heart rates continue to be stable, she may be placed inside an incubator crib, also called an isolette. This enclosed crib is designed to keep your baby warm until she demonstrates that she can regulate her body temperature and stay warm on her own. (Isolette seems an unfortunate name for a baby bed, even one specially made for premature infants. It is not physiologically good for baby to be isolated from the loving touch of his parents.)

Infants who are very premature. If your baby was born 8 weeks or more before your due date, or if your baby has immediate difficulties with breathing, he may be receiving quite a bit of high-tech care when you first visit the nursery. Seeing your newborn baby receiving full intensive care can be frightening for any parent. You may feel reluctant to get close to baby until he is more stable. You may be scared to touch and caress him when he appears to be in such a fragile state. But take a deep breath and look past all the machines and wires at the tiny person underneath — your precious child. It is okay to touch him (the nurses will help you with this), to lay your hand on his back or head, to tell him that you love him. Although you won't be able to see it at first, your baby will benefit from your touch. And this early contact will call forth the parent in you and help you cope with your emotions.

I was not adequately prepared to see my baby with all the tubes and monitors and the eye coverings.

PROFILE OF A PREEMIE

What your baby looks like depends upon her degree of prematurity. If your baby was born 8 or more weeks premature, there will be noticeable differences between how your baby looks and how a full-term infant looks. You may initially be shocked to see how tiny your baby is, but after you get a chance to look her over and notice that everything is there — ten fingers and ten toes! — you'll marvel at how completely formed she is. These tiny body parts are just waiting to grow.

Here are the most common differences between full-term and premature newborns:

Skin. Preemies lack the thick layer of plump baby fat that is stored just under the skin during the last few weeks of pregnancy, so their skin often appears wrinkled, as if it doesn't yet fit. It is thin and transparent, compared with that of a full-term baby. You may even be able to see the lacelike arteries and veins just underneath the surface. The younger the baby, the thinner the skin and the more reddish-purple its color. Even premature babies of dark-skinned parents often have reddish-pink skin. In extremely premature babies (28 weeks and below), the skin may look especially thin, shiny, and fragile.

Head. A preemie's head appears large in proportion to the rest of her body. And, since much of the body's heat is lost from the head, expect her head to be covered with a little cap during most of her hospital stay. Even some full-term babies wear these caps.

Hands and feet. Because of the lack of fat, the fingers look slender and long in relation to those tiny but adorable hands. Fingernails and toenails may be barely perceptible. By the time baby reaches full maturity, the nails are likely to grow to the ends of the fingers and toes. The more premature the baby, the less developed are the creases on the soles of the feet. In fact, neonatal care specialists use the development of these sole creases as one indication of the baby's degree of prematurity.

Hair. Baby will have a soft, fuzzy layer of hair over most of her body, especially on the upper back, shoulders, and arms. The younger the preemie, the fuzzier it will be. Called lanugo, this hair may help keep baby warm in the early weeks. Your baby may shed much of this preemie hair within a few weeks. In the last four weeks of gestation, this baby hair becomes thicker and more silken.

Eyes. Your baby may keep her eyes closed much of the time because babies' eyes are sensitive to light, especially if they are extremely premature (28 weeks or below).

Ears. Ear cartilage that gives ears their firm appearance develops around week 35 of pregnancy. Before that, expect your baby's ears to be floppy and sometimes folded over.

Genitalia. Preemies of less than 34 weeks' gestation may have underdeveloped genitalia. A boy baby's testes may or may not be descended, and the labia of a premature girl may be small. Premature baby girls often have a tag of tissue, called a hymen tag, protruding from the vagina. This extra tissue will eventually disappear. Like the sole creases, the genitalia give doctors clues to the degree of baby's prematurity.

Muscle tone. The more premature your baby, the more "floppy" her muscle tone. Very premature babies tend to have very loose muscle tone.

His tiny buns looked like deflated balloons.

Rib cage. Baby's rib cage and breastbone are soft and pliable, and the chest may appear to cave in with each breath. Termed retractions, these chest movements are normal to some degree, but if extreme, they may be an indication of breathing difficulties.

Arms and legs. When preemies are placed on their backs, their arms lie straight out at their sides, and their legs are bent open like little frogs' legs. (A more mature baby will hold his arms and legs in a flexed position, pulled close to the body.) Baby's limbs will appear slender in relation to the rest of her body. These skinny arms and legs, along with a protruding abdomen, may make your preemie look like a malnourished baby. Don't let this scare you. Your baby will fill out within a few weeks as she begins to build muscles and store baby fat.

Take the time to explore and become comfortable with your baby's tiny body. Take pictures, so that you have a before and after record of her time in the NICU. Your baby will change rapidly over the next several weeks.

ALL WIRED UP FOR INTENSIVE CARE

The machines and wires surrounding your baby will be less intimidating if you know what they are and what they do. Ask the nurses to explain anything you don't understand. Here is an overview of what you can expect, depending on how critically ill your baby is.

Ventilator. The ventilator (also called a respirator) breathes for your baby until she is ready to breathe on her own. The ventilator pumps air and oxygen into your baby's lungs through a tube called an endotrachial, or ET, tube. The tube is inserted through your baby's mouth or nose down into her windpipe. (Because it passes through the vocal cords, your baby's cries will not be audible.) This tube may be secured by a piece of tape on baby's nose and cheeks.

Radiant warmer. Sometimes right after birth, babies are placed in an open bassinet with a warming device above it. This setup is often used for the first few hours, while baby's condition is being assessed by the doctors and nurses and tests and procedures are being done. It is also used during critical times, when rapid access to your baby may be needed.

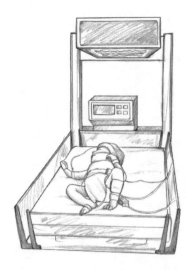

Isolette. Also called an incubator, the isolette will be your baby's bed for a while. The isolette keeps your baby from getting cold. Because your baby has not yet grown a layer of insulating fat beneath her skin, it's very easy for her body to lose heat. A small button, called a temperature probe, placed above your baby's tummy is connected to a wire that leads to a thermostat. The thermostat automatically adjusts the temperature of the isolette to keep your baby's body temperature stable. You will notice that one side of the isolette is a door with two "portholes" in it that allow you and the nurses to reach in and care for and comfort your baby. The door can be unlatched and opened, allow-

ing the nurse to take your baby out of the isolette when necessary. Get comfortable with putting your hands through these portholes so you can change your baby's diapers, stroke her skin, and comfort and bond with her. It is generally okay to take baby out of the incubator for short periods of time for some extra physical contact. Your baby's nurse will help you with this.

Pulse oximeter. You may see a tiny sensor taped to your baby's hand or foot. It measures the percentage of oxygen in her blood.

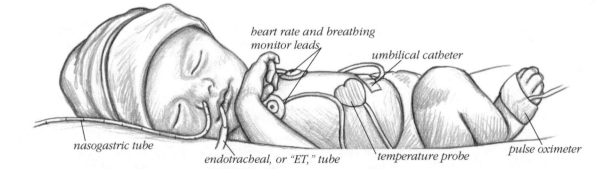

heart rate and breathing monitor leads

umbilical catheter

nasogastric tube

endotracheal, or "ET," tube

temperature probe

pulse oximeter

Heart rate and breathing monitor. You will notice wires taped to your baby's chest and legs. These detect her heartbeat and respirations and display the information on a monitor.

Tubes and lines. Intravenous lines (also called catheters) may be placed in your baby's hand, foot, or umbilical vein to deliver fluids and medications into her bloodstream. For the first few days, your baby may have another line inserted into her umbilical artery, which allows the nurses to take frequent blood samples painlessly. Large veins in the scalp are another convenient place for an IV. Regard the tubes and lines as a sort of time-line of your preemie's progress. As the number of tubes gets fewer and the IV lines get smaller, you will know your baby is finding her way in the world outside the womb.

Nasogastric or orogastric tube. A thin, flexible tube inserted through your baby's nose down into her stomach is called a nasogastric tube. If this tube is placed through the mouth into the stomach, it is called an orogastric tube. While this tube will eventually be used to feed your baby, its initial purpose is to suction swallowed air and acid out of the stomach when baby is having difficulty breathing. Babies swallow a lot of air, which distends the stomach, presses on the diaphragm, and compromises breathing.

Blood pressure monitor. A tiny inflatable blood pressure cuff is wrapped around your baby's arm or leg and may be left in place so that the nurse can take your baby's blood pressure without constantly putting it on and taking it off.

Nasal canula. Tiny prongs are inserted into your baby's nostrils to deliver humidified oxygen for easier breathing.

Oxygen hood. A clear plastic tent that fits around your baby's head may be used to deliver warm, moist oxygen. This makes breathing easier for babies who are not on ventilators.

Dr. Bob advises: Keep a keen eye on all the goings-on around your baby. If your parental instinct tells you something is not right, question it. Not only does asking about monitor readings help you learn about this technology, but you owe it to your baby to be her advocate. Mother's and Father's eyes will see things that no one else sees.

FINDING FRIENDS IN THE NICU — A TALE OF TWO FAMILIES

As you sit next to your new baby, take a look around the room. This will be your baby's home, possibly for several weeks. Do you withdraw into your own little world, feeling lost and alone, ignoring

---

APPRECIATE THE MECHANICAL WOMB

While it's understandably upsetting to see your tiny baby "all wired up to those weird machines," think of them as a "womb" that will shelter and protect your baby for a few more weeks.

everything and everyone else? Or do you make yourself at home, get to know the medical staff, and develop friendships with the nurses and other parents? We periodically visit our patients in our local NICU, and in our experience, the way parents personally answer these two questions has a dramatic impact on their time in the NICU. Handling the initial stress of their baby's early days, learning to cope with the challenges, interacting with the NICU staff, and rejoicing in the successes of their baby all shape parents' overall impressions and memories of this time. Our patients share with us their experiences. Some look back on these weeks as a challenging but growing time with their baby. Others remember it as a fearful, invasive, negative experience that they wish to forget.

Here is a common scenario that we have seen many of our patients go through: Baby is born suddenly at 30 weeks' gestation. The little one immediately develops breathing difficulties and is rushed to the NICU. The baby requires intensive care, including assisted ventilation for breathing. Dad follows baby up to the NICU and feels helpless and confused about everything that is being done to his baby, although, as a father, he does want to understand what his baby needs and why. A nurse notices Dad's uncertainty and interest and takes a few minutes to explain to him what all the monitors, tubes, and wires are for. She encourages him to stay by the baby's bedside, to touch and bond with baby while the medical staff do their job. Now, here is typically where the various personality types and different abilities to cope with stress and face uncertain situations come into play.

Scenario #1. Some of our patients who are able to cope better have experiences that continue positively.

Dad trusts the medical staff to take good care of his baby and concentrates on baby's tiny features and fuzzy hair, so that he can tell his wife about their baby when he goes back to her room. When both Mom and Dad visit the NICU together, Dad gives her a simple explanation of the different pieces of equipment. The baby's nurse provides some more information and shows Mom the best way to touch and stroke her newborn. The parents are uncomfortable with some of the medical procedures but accept the nurses' explanations and reassurances. Over the next few days, they become more comfortable with the medical routine as they feed, hold, and observe their baby. The numerous daily monitor alarms and IV beeps don't bother the parents, because they've learned these are routine and will be attended to by their nurse, whom they've grown to trust. They aren't necessarily thrilled with all the blood tests and procedures, but they know these are important. They make some suggestions about baby's care, which are listened to and accommodated. They also get to know the parents around them and provide mutual support. When baby is ready to go home, Mom and Dad leave the NICU with new friendships and the feeling that they were supported and loved, and that their baby received outstanding care. They feel reassured that they can call the staff for advice during those anxious first weeks at home.

Scenario #2. Some of our patients who find it more challenging to deal with stress and the uncertainty of having a preemie relate a much different experience to us.

Dad follows baby up to the NICU and feels helpless and confused about everything that is being done to his baby. He is a person who is used to being in control and knowing everything about everything, so he begins asking for explanations from the nursing staff about everything that they are doing "to" his baby. The medical staff are accustomed to being around worried parents, and the doctors and nurses do their best to patiently explain everything to him and to encourage him to touch and comfort his baby. But Dad isn't satisfied and wants to speak to the doctor *again*.

Mom joins Dad in the NICU, and they both stay by their baby's bedside. Dad describes in graphic detail everything they've done "to" (not "for") the baby. A nurse comes to draw blood, but Dad doesn't want his baby "poked" again and demands that the nurse check with the doctor to see if the tests are really necessary. An X-ray technician brings a portable X-ray machine to take an X-ray of the baby's lungs. Mom is worried about exposing her baby to the radiation and wants to speak with the doctor about whether the X-ray is safe or not. The baby's IV stops working and the nurse needs to put in another one. Dad gets angry because he (naturally) hates to see his baby in pain from IV needles. The NICU nurses and doctor try to be patient and sensitive with the parents, but even after several days in the NICU, the parents continue to question everything done for their baby. Every time a monitor beeps or an alarm sounds, Dad demands immediate attention and protests if a nurse doesn't immediately rush to check on their baby.

Word spreads among the NICU staff that these parents are "high maintenance" and sometimes downright rude and difficult to deal with. The NICU staff are used to helping all types of parents, and they continue to patiently provide quality medical care to the baby, but the parents withdraw into their own worried world. They research their baby's care on the Internet, but they fail to develop a trusting relationship with the nurses and doctors. This makes it difficult for the staff to reassure these parents and help them understand their baby's progress. When their baby is discharged, the family leaves the NICU with only memories of a difficult beginning that they try to put behind them.

In both these scenarios, the babies got the expert care they needed. But families who approach this stressful time as the second couple did, face a far more emotionally stressful few weeks.

Parents are right to look out for their baby's well-being, to keep asking questions until they understand everything to their own satisfaction. Part of your job as a parent is to make sure your baby is getting the best medical care possible.

Yet, it is important for you as a parent and as a part of the medical team caring for your baby to find a balance. Treat the medical staff with respect, and they will respect you in turn. Trusting the doctors and nurses to do their jobs well will free you up to stay positive and do the job that no one else can do as well as you — loving and caring for your baby.

Dr. Jim advises: When talking to parents of NICU grads, ask to see "before and after" pictures. You

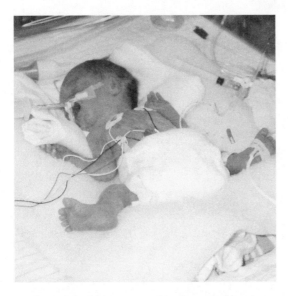
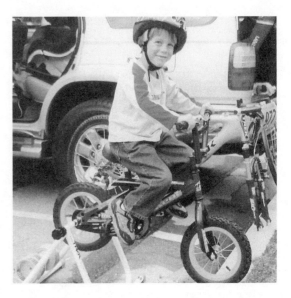

"Before and after" pictures of Sterling von Hartmann.

will see that the tiny baby who began life in an isolette just a few years ago is now riding a tricycle through the park at break-neck speed. Evidence like this reassures you that in all likelihood your baby will grow up to be just fine.

CONSULT OTHER NICU PARENTS

Get to know some of the "veterans" — parents who have been with their babies in the NICU for several weeks. They have not only "been there, done that," but they are still there and are still doing that. They can truly empathize with what you are feeling. Also, the hospital may have a list of parents of NICU graduates who have volunteered to talk to other parents. These supportive volunteers are often very good at translating technical medical jargon into parent-friendly language.

BE NICE TO THE NURSES

Show your appreciation for the nurses. Let them know they're making a difference. Perhaps you could write a note from your baby addressed "To my nurse" and leave it on the incubator. If friends and neighbors are bringing you goodies, share these treats with the staff. Send photos and cards after you leave the hospital. The medical staff really appreciate hearing how their charges are doing after they leave the hospital.

I owe a debt to the women and men who saved my son's life and who cared for him every day. I thank them for their care and medical knowledge, and especially for the little things, like the Mother's Day card they made for me with Will's footprint.

◆

Bring treats for the nurses. I know this sounds nuts, but I hoped that maybe, since I brought them some chocolates for the night shift, they would be sweeter to my baby when I wasn't there.

Besides you, the person who will spend by far the most time with your baby is your baby's nurse. NICU nurses generally work in twelve- or eight-hour shifts. You will get to know several nurses during your stay, and you will probably see the same nurses caring for your baby day to day.

I really liked the nurses who gave me a lot of details, like how many messy diapers my baby had, how many wet ones, how much she ate, etc. Knowing all those little details helped me get to know my baby and feel more involved.

Get behind the eyes of the staff. There will be days when they seem abrupt, hurried, or aloof, but remember, they have a difficult job to do. They are often overworked and under a lot of stress themselves. See how you can help. A well-timed gift or a caring word does wonders, such as, "I know you're in a hurry. I'll ask the question again when you have more time."

Laughter is the best medicine. Leave little humorous notes around the isolette for you and the nurses to read.

Take the time to get to know your nurses by name. Let them know that you are an interested, involved, and educated parent who wants to help. Respect your nurses, and they in turn will show you the support and respect you want. They will be your most valuable allies in helping you stay involved in your baby's care.

I appreciated that some of the nurses made signs for him, like "Watch me

grow — I'm 4 pounds now!" One nurse made "cool" sunglasses for his eye covers while he was under the bililight.

An important person in the NICU whom you should get to know by name is the *charge nurse.* This nurse is in charge of all the nurses in the unit on a shift. There will be different charge nurses on different shifts. If you can, take the time to say hello to the charge nurse every time you are in the NICU. Knowing the nurses by name and helping them get to know you means you will have someone you can turn to if any problems arise that are not solved to your satisfaction.

When my favorite nurse, Annette, first took my baby out of the isolette and handed him to me, she said, "See, he knows who his mommy is." That set tears in motion again. What an amazing feeling! I waited thirty-six hours to hold my newborn, and he was worth every minute of that wait.

NICU RULES YOU SHOULD KNOW

For the sake of your baby and the other babies and families, there are rules and etiquette to be observed in the NICU.

Wash your hands, please! On your first visit to the unit, a nurse will walk you through a "scrub-in" routine that you will repeat many times during your baby's stay in the NICU. You may feel like a surgeon preparing for surgery: you will wash your hands for a specified amount of time with antibacterial soap before entering the unit. The medical staff must do the same thing. This procedure is designed to keep germs out of the NICU. The NICU is not a sterile environment, but rules about hand washing go a long way toward protecting your baby and other babies in the unit from infection and illness. Respect this rule and follow the procedure every time you enter the unit. Most NICUs do not require parents to wear hospital gowns over their clothing anymore, since gown wearing hasn't been shown to reduce infection rates.

Know visiting policies. Each NICU has different policies about visitors. Ask about these as soon as possible if other family members want to visit your baby. Some units will not allow small children to visit under any circumstances. Theoretically, kids tend to harbor cold germs generally more readily than adults do, and a simple cold virus can wreak havoc if it spreads through a neonatal nursery. Yet more hospitals are now welcoming siblings to visit their tiny brother or sister, provided they take the same sanitary precautions as their parents.

Most NICUs allow parents to visit at any time and to spend as much time as they like with their baby. You may find that the staff will encourage you to take breaks from time to time, to go home and get some sleep, and especially to go get something good to eat at mealtimes. For parents who want to spend every second with baby, these friendly suggestions can get annoying. The nurses mean well, and they have seen many parents wear themselves out by trying to be on watch 24/7. Don't automatically reject their advice.

Know when to leave. Try not to be upset if you are asked to periodically leave your baby's bedside, especially during certain procedures, such as drawing blood or inserting a tube into your baby's airway, or during a doctor's rounds. While

you may feel a bit put out by being excluded from these inner circles, there are legitimate reasons for this. The staff performing the procedure may feel more self-conscious or distracted in your presence, and that might interfere with the accuracy and ease of a procedure. The staff may feel that a certain procedure may upset you, especially if they think you already have enough stress to deal with. Make each decision to stay or go a situation-by-situation judgment call. If you want to stay during a certain procedure, ask. Assure the staff that you have command over your emotions and will not interfere. If you don't want to stay, leave gracefully. Many parents feel it's very comforting for their baby to have them there stroking him and singing to him during a procedure such as the insertion of an IV. In time, you'll gradually learn when to stay to lend a helping hand and when it's best to leave.

There are two specific times when the medical staff will ask you to briefly leave the unit. During nursing shift changes (every eight or twelve hours), the nurses will discuss the care of your baby and the other babies nearby. In order to respect the medical privacy of all the families involved, visitors will be asked to leave during this half hour. Another such time is morning rounds. During this hour, all the doctors on the unit will move from patient to patient and openly discuss the baby's care with the rest of the health care team. Of course, it would not be appropriate for parents of one baby to hear the details of another baby's care. The doctors and nurses also need to be able to openly discuss complications and treatment options without concern for those who might overhear. Take advantage of these respites and grab a bite to eat and talk with other parents.

Be prepared to be rushed a bit if the nurses are changing shifts and you are in the middle of a feeding. Nurses will want to wind up their reports, making the transition to the next nurse go smoothly. That just goes with the NICU territory.

If you have questions about NICU policies, ask the head nurse for clarification. Then, if a conflict arises between what you think unit policy is and what is actually happening, you can say, "I'm sorry, but I understood the policy was . . ." This is a nonconfrontational way to question your baby's care or the unit's rules. There may be a particular reason why your baby's care does not follow the standard policy, and your baby's nurse will then explain it to you. Or the nurse may need to clarify the policy with the charge nurse and then report to you. Veteran nurses expect you to be your baby's advocate, but they also appreciate being treated with respect.

NICU COMMUNICATION TIPS

You'll be talking — and listening — to NICU staff members many times during the coming days and weeks. Good two-way communication is critical to your feeling comfortable parenting your baby in this stressful time. Here are some communication courtesies that will help not only you but also the NICU staff provide high-quality care for your baby.

Communicate your comfort level. Let the nurses know the degree to which you want to be involved with your baby's care. Remember, they have your and your baby's best interests in mind. They don't want to force you to do more than you are ready to do, but they do want to help and support you as you become involved with your baby.

If the nurses know you want to know details, they'll oblige. In fact, better nurses realize this and will often fill your ears with cute little details as soon as you enter the NICU.

Don't be afraid to ask questions. The doctors and nursing staff want you to know what's going on with your baby. They welcome your concern and curiosity. Don't worry about asking "dumb questions." You are the parent, and your baby is premature. Enough said.

Every morning, as soon as I arrived at the hospital, I was completely updated on my baby's condition and how his night was. I appreciated that.

Ask whom to ask. Most of what you are told about your baby will come from the neonatal nurses because they are there all the time. If you wish to talk directly to the doctor, ask to do so. In your initial consultation with the doctor, ask to whom you should direct most of your questions. Find out the best way to contact this person.

"Could you please explain . . ." If the doctor or nurse explains a procedure or medical occurrence in words that are too technical for you to understand, say so. It's okay to say, "I don't understand those terms. Could you explain this to me in plain language?" Another helpful strategy is to repeat what you have just been told in your own words: "So you are saying that my baby's breathing difficulties are the result of . . ." This gives the doctor or nurse an opportunity to check your understanding of what was said.

Don't hesitate to ask the doctor or nurse to repeat a medical explanation. They realize that you're feeling so much stress that you are unlikely to retain much of what was said the first time. They're used to repeating things until they sink in. You'll find that many have infinite patience — otherwise, they wouldn't be in that profession.

Ask about telephone calls. When you are at home, you will want to call the NICU to check on your baby. Usually parents have access to the NICU nurses by phone twenty-four hours a day. However, some times are better than others for phone calls. Ask about the best time to call. Keep your phone calls brief and to the point. You may just need a periodic update. Discourage friends and relatives from calling the NICU directly for an update on your baby. It's better if they get information directly from you. The NICU staff are very busy, and their time is better spent caring for babies than talking to relatives on the telephone.

Dr. Jim advises: If you yourself don't want to talk to a lot of people, share your baby news with one designated individual and then let others know that they can call him or her for information. Or, periodically record a baby update on your home answering machine or e-mail text and photos.

Remind the staff. Sometimes a doctor or nurse may downplay a potential problem by saying something like, "It's no big deal, we'll discuss it later." Yet it may be a big deal to you. Don't wonder and worry. Ask for more information, either right away or the next time you talk with the doctor. Remind the caregiver, "You said you would tell me about it later."

I was told that she had a grade I brain bleed that "usually doesn't add up to anything but needs to be checked again." No one ever mentioned it again, and I kept wondering what they meant by "needs to be checked again."

Volunteer. Some NICUs are understaffed, or the nurses may seem to be having a hectic day for some reason. They'll welcome your help. You might say something like this: "I know you're busy, so please tell me what I can do to help, and have patience with me."

Ask to take over as much of your baby's care as possible, such as bathing, feeding, changing, etc. It helps the nurses to know the level of care you want to give. They always walk a fine line between telling you to do too much and asking you to do too little.

Stay positive. It is especially important to have a positive attitude during the first few days of critical care. This is not a time to lecture the staff about what you don't want done to your baby. Staying upbeat and relaxed in your communication with staff indirectly helps your baby's care. Everyone does a better job in a positive atmosphere.

Speak up when you are happy with your baby's care.

Plan ahead. If you know ahead of time that you may deliver early, either because of medical complications or because you are pregnant with multiples, prepare yourself and become familiar with the NICU before you need it. It's hard to learn the ropes when you are sleep deprived, recovering from giving birth, and grief stricken at being separated from your baby. Familiarize yourself with the NICU environment and available resources before you need them. Rehearse and repeatedly imagine the scene and mentally and emotionally prepare for the fact that your baby will be taken away from you and placed in the NICU after delivery. Tour the NICU and meet some of the staff. You can probably get a staff nurse to give you a private tour.

Respect different approaches. What you hear from one member of the medical staff may be different from what you hear from another. One person may go into great detail about the risks of a procedure or the chances of your preemie experiencing long-term problems. Another may minimize possible complications and calmly reassure you that everything is going to be just fine. Do these two individuals really have such different opinions about your baby's condition? Probably not. They just have different views about how to talk with parents.

One school of thought believes in informing parents of all the possibilities, gruesome as they may be, so they are prepared and not surprised if the worst comes to pass. If baby sails through without problems, parents are relieved and overjoyed. The opposing school of thought says, Why burden parents with worries about complications that may never happen? Why let fears about the future rob parents of hope in the present? There is merit in both of these approaches, and the one that health professionals adopt may have more to do with their individual personality than their training.

Probably the best approach for most parents lies somewhere in the middle. Remember, if the doctor doesn't mention all the possible problems your baby may have down the road, it doesn't mean that he or she doesn't know about them. If there are issues that are worrying you, be sure to ask about them, even if the doctor doesn't bring them up. And if a particular doctor's enumeration of all the possible problems your preemie faces leaves you too frightened to cope, don't go to that individual with your questions. Find someone more reassuring to talk with.

Initially, I was annoyed at the inconsistency and different levels of sharing of the staff, but then I realized that people are different. I learned where I could get the best advice and answers to my questions.

WHO'S WHO IN THE NICU

Get to know all the special people caring for your baby in the special care nursery. Treat them well, as they will be part of your extended medical family for the next few days or weeks. Depending on the level of the NICU and whether or not it is a university's teaching hospital, your baby will be cared for by some or all of the following professionals.

Neonatologist. This doctor is in charge of the unit and all the babies. He or she is a pediatrician with an extra three years of training in neonatology, the care of newborns. A large university teaching hospital may have several neonatologists on staff. They each take turns working as the physician in charge of the unit. You may hear the staff refer to your baby's neonatologist as the attending physician, the one who sees your baby daily and personally supervises your baby's care.

I tried to be my baby's constant companion when everything else could change in a minute. I wanted to be the one person who would always be there for him.

Neonatology fellow. He or she is a pediatrician who is in a three-year training program in neonatology. There may be more than one fellow working in the unit, and the fellows take turns spending the night in the hospital so that a physician is immediately available for any emergencies. Because he or she is spending all day and some nights in the unit, the neonatology fellow will be intimately involved in the details of your baby's care.

Neonatal nurse practitioner. Also known as NNPs, neonatal nurse practitioners have had advanced training in newborn special care. They act as assistants to the neonatologist and can carry out many of the duties of a neonatologist, such as ordering medications and performing procedures.

Pediatric resident. This doctor has finished medical school and is now in a three-year training program to become a pediatrician. Residents typically spend three months working in a neonatal nursery during their residency. There are several residents assigned to the unit during any given month, and they take turns spending the night in the hospital to help the fellow or nurse practitioner with any emergencies. The resident will pay close attention to every detail about your baby and report to the fellow and attending physician. As a team, these doctors will make decisions together about your baby's medical care.

A smaller, nonteaching community hospital may not have pediatric residents or fellows. Instead, your baby's care will be supervised by a few neonatologists who each work several days a week and take turns staying overnight. They may be assisted by a nurse practitioner.

Neonatal nurse. These VIPs in your baby's care will be at your baby's bedside 24/7. They are responsible for carrying out the doctor's orders, giving medication, feeding your baby, bathing her, weighing her, changing her diapers, evaluating the monitor readings, and generally keeping an eye on her and watching for changes in her condition. Of all the members of the medical team, you will probably get to know the nurses best, since they are the ones who will spend the most time at your baby's bedside. Depending on the length of your baby's NICU stay, you may get your honorary degree as a "neonatal nurse."

The nurses became like family. Not only were the doctors and nurses skilled, but I got the feeling they really cared about my baby.

Besides the nurses and doctors, there are several other medical personnel who will be involved in your baby's care.

Respiratory therapist. Respiratory therapists are experts in ventilators and all the other apparatus that assist your baby's breathing. They come by regularly to check the ventilator and the associated tubing.

Lactation consultant. NICUs have a lactation consultant on staff to help you learn how to pump and store your breast milk, assist you with any pumping difficulties, and help you get started with breastfeeding as soon as baby is ready.

Blood drawing technician. These technicians come through the unit every morning to draw blood samples according to the doctors' orders. The nurses and doctors may also draw blood.

Social worker. NICUs have social workers on staff to help you adapt to your new life as the parent of a preemie, listen to and try to address any of your concerns, and assist you with insurance or financial issues. They act as a liaison between the NICU and the outside world. When it is time for your baby to be discharged, they will help you with any special needs or special equipment, arrange follow-up doctor's appointments, and make sure you are comfortable taking baby home. The social workers are there to turn to anytime you need another sympathetic ear.

Occupational therapist. If your baby has any special developmental issues that require closer observation and therapy, occupational therapists are available in the unit. If, for example, your premature baby is having difficulty learning to feed, an OT may routinely check on what's going on and offer suggestions.

Nutritionist. Many NICUs use nutritionists to periodically assess a baby's growth and nutritional requirements and make sure these are being met.

Last, but not least, are *other parents.* Those who have been with their baby in the NICU for a while are one of your most valuable resources. Ask your nurse to introduce you to a veteran mom or dad who would be willing to spend some time with you. Have lunch with other parents. Ask them to share their feelings and experiences with you. Relying on support from other parents, and offering your support in turn to others, will make your experience in the NICU more positive.

Dr. Bob advises: No one can completely prepare you for parenting a preemie. It requires on-the-job training. Yet, like any "job," it comes with training manuals (books such as this one), support staff (the NICU personnel), supportive coworkers (your spouse), and colleagues in your field (other parents of babies in the NICU). Take advantage of all these resources as you master your job as the parent of a preemie.

CONFESSIONS OF A NICU DOCTOR

The two years I (Dr. Bill) spent getting extra training in neonatology and the four years that followed, when I worked as an associate ward chief in the NICU, were among the most challenging years of my professional career. Parents of preemies talk about being on a roller-coaster ride; doctors and nurses on the NICU staff experience the same kinds of extreme ups and downs.

NICU SPEAK

As you sit by your baby's bedside, you will hear the nurses and doctors around you speaking what seems like a foreign language. Here's a quick guide to the most commonly used "NICU speak" that will help you make better sense of everything you see and hear. For an explanation of these terms and a more complete list of terms, refer to the glossary on page 229.

As and Bs: periods of apnea and brady-cardia (slower breathing and heart rate respectively)

ABG: arterial blood gases

Bagging or **bagged:** pumping air into baby's lungs with a rubber or plastic breathing bag

Bili: bilirubin

Blow-by: giving baby a small amount of oxygen through a tube pointed toward baby's nose

Central line: an IV placed in the arm, groin, or chest that extends up into a large blood vessel; different from a peripheral IV line, which goes only an inch or two into a small vein

Chem strip: blood sugar level

CPAP: continuous positive airway pressure

De-satting or **desaturation:** a drop in oxygen levels in baby's blood-stream

Drip: IV fluid from a bag containing fluids

ET tube: endotracheal tube

Hyperal: hyperalimentation

Is and Os: the amount of fluids (IV and feeds) baby takes *in* compared to how much baby pees and poops *out*

Intubate: to insert an ET tube into baby's lungs

Leads: monitor wires taped to baby's skin; baby's monitor can set off the alarm due to what nurses call "loose leads"

NG tube: nasogastric tube

NPO: abbreviation for the Latin term *nil per os,* meaning "nothing by mouth"

O2 sats: oxygen saturation — the level of oxygen in baby's bloodstream, as in "baby's sats are stable"

Platelets: the type of blood cell that creates blood clots and scabs to stop bleeding

Pulse ox: short for pulse oximeter, an oxygen saturation monitor

Sepsis: a serious infection in the blood-stream that can affect various organs and cause serious complications; treated with antibiotics and intensive care

TPN: total parenteral nutrition

Urine dip: a dipstick test of baby's urine; used to monitor baby's hydra-tion status

Vent: ventilator

When I worked in the NICU, I never knew what kind of day it would be. I would make the same drive to the hospital every morning, park in the same place, scrub my hands, don my gown, and enter another world, where nothing was predictable and nothing would be the same as it was yesterday. Some days I would enter the unit in the morning to make rounds and hear that it had been a good night. All the babies had survived, some were weaned off ventilators, and some had gained weight. Other days I would open the door to the NICU and know immediately that the night before had been rough and the day that lay ahead of me was going to be difficult.

The NICU doctor makes life-or-death decisions daily. Many of these are judgment calls that must be made quickly. When everything turns out well, the doctor is almost as happy as the baby's parents (maybe more so, since we are more aware of all the things that can go wrong). Yet, a NICU doctor must understand the fact that years of experience and the best clinical judgment do not guarantee good outcomes every time. NICU staff members have to live with the decisions that turn out well and the ones that don't. And everything happens so fast.

Just like everyone else, NICU doctors and nurses have days when they're tired or sad and days when they're feeling energetic and upbeat. They have days when they enjoy coming to work and days when they'd rather go sailing. What keeps them going is the incredibly good feeling that comes from providing expert care that will make the lives of most babies in the NICU — and their parents — better. Doctors especially are expected to be positive and confident, sometimes unrealistically so, as they set the tone for the care provided by the entire NICU staff.

Years and years of training in neonatology do not prepare physicians for the hardest part of their job: dealing with parents who are going through one of the most difficult periods of their lives. Neonatologists have to learn this part of the profession on the job. There were days when I felt that all I did was deliver bad news to parents who had been hoping for the best. Professional ethics demanded that I be honest with the parents of my patients, but I would want to hedge a bit. I was a parent, too, and I knew that hope was what kept parents going.

Doctors learn to understand that parents will sometimes dump their own frustrations on the medical staff. Many times, when parents ask questions, the doctor can't answer them, at least not in a way that satisfies parents' need to believe that everything is going to be okay. Sometimes doctors can get behind the eyes of the parents of their patients and empathize with all they are going through. Sometimes doctors know that even though they are doing their best, it is not enough to satisfy parents who love their baby intensely and are very worried, especially if their baby is not making the progress everyone was hoping to see.

At the end of a shift in the NICU, the doctors get to go home, back to a more predictable world. The burdens of the day remain, but buried beneath the exhaustion and frustration is the feeling that babies and parents are mostly better off because of what they said and did that day. That's what keeps NICU doctors going.

Neonatology 101 — A Primer for Parents of Preemies

IN OVER THIRTY YEARS of working with parents of preemies (POPs) and their babies, we have learned a valuable lesson: the more parents understand the details particular to their baby's condition, and the medical procedures necessary as a result of these "preemie quirks," the better able they are to cope, to participate in their baby's care, and to get to know and feel comfortable with their baby. In the previous chapter, you learned a lot about your baby's medical care. Here's a second and larger helping of information that you need to know. Don't be afraid to learn more about your baby. The more you understand, the less you will worry.

Prematurity is not itself a disease. Yet, being born prematurely does present a variety of medical challenges in each of the baby's delicate body systems. Preemie care is aimed at reproducing, as closely as possible, the conditions your baby would have found in the womb had she remained there to term. The greatest challenges are supplying oxygen and nutrition to baby. In the womb, these were received through the umbilical cord directly into the bloodstream, and the lungs and intestines were not required. Now, the only way to give baby oxygen is through lungs that are not yet ready to be used. Efforts are made to make baby's lungs quickly adjust to life outside the womb and make oxygen absorption possible. In the NICU, baby initially receives IV nutrition through the umbilical vein, just like in the womb. The transition to milk feedings requires that baby's intestines mature first.

In this chapter, we will explain how the transition to regular breathing and milk feedings is achieved. We'll go over how the equipment works, why it is used, and what tests are routinely done to evaluate your baby's progress. Of course, your own baby's situation may differ from this general description of preemie problems, but we hope that with this background information and your doctors' and nurses' explanations, you will fully understand what is going on with your baby.

Try to feel like a mommy even though sometimes you feel more like a nurse.

A WOMB WITH A VIEW

A mother of a preemie once told us that she was able to think of the NICU in more positive terms once she realized that she had the privilege of watching her baby grow in a sort of outside womb. This view of your baby's caregiving environment can help you to overcome the feelings of loss, detachment, and displacement that are only natural when your baby is born too soon. If you think of her home in the NICU as another kind of womb, one in which you can continue to protect and care for her, you will feel closer and more attached to your baby. True, you are missing out on the last weeks of pregnancy, but being able to watch her grow in this outside womb is another kind of miracle.

RESPIRATORY SYSTEM

Most babies born after 36 weeks of pregnancy do not have any significant breathing problems. The earlier your baby is born, the more likely he or she is to require assistance in breathing until the lungs mature. Why don't preemie lungs work well? Lung tissue is made up of millions of tiny round pockets called alveoli. These alveoli expand as the air moves in. Inside the alveoli is a thin layer of liquid called surfactant, which helps the alveoli open up. Surfactant is essential for the exchange of oxygen and carbon dioxide between the lungs and the bloodstream. Premature babies lack enough surfactant in the lungs, and as a result, the alveoli in their lungs don't open up well and don't trap oxygen well enough for it to be efficiently absorbed into the bloodstream. This breathing problem is called Respiratory Distress Syndrome (RDS). (Sometimes if a mother knows ahead of time that she will be delivering her baby prematurely, obstetricians will give her steroid medications to help baby's lungs make more surfactant and mature more quickly.)

Oxygen. Neonatologists use several different strategies to ensure that your baby is getting enough oxygen into her bloodstream during the time that her lungs are immature and she is not making enough surfactant to breathe well. One way to improve your baby's oxygen absorption is to increase the concentration of oxygen in the air she is breathing. Normal air in a room is about 21 percent oxygen. Babies can receive as much as 100 percent oxygen in extreme cases. How does your doctor know how much oxygen your baby needs? An oxygen saturation monitor (also called a pulse ox) is taped to your baby's hand or foot. It measures the oxygen levels in your baby's blood by shining a light through the skin. Healthy babies should be able to maintain an oxygen saturation (termed an O2 sat) level of 95 to 100 percent while breathing normal room air. Your doctor or nurse will give your baby enough oxygen to maintain an oxygen saturation of 90 percent or higher. There are several ways this is achieved:

• *Nasal canula.* A thin plastic tube is taped to your baby's upper lip and two short prongs point up into the baby's nose to deliver oxygen.

- *Oxygen hood.* A plastic dome is placed over baby's upper body and humid oxygen-enriched air is blown in through a tube. The air baby breathes has a higher oxygen concentration.
- *Blow-by oxygen.* This is the least invasive way to deliver oxygen to baby. An oxygen hose is simply pointed toward baby's face. This is often used if baby needs oxygen only at special times, for example, during feedings.
- *Nasal Continuous Positive Airway Pressure (Nasal CPAP).* This technique involves a tube placed in baby's nose. Oxygen under pressure is continuously blown through baby's nose and down into the lungs. This pressure helps keep the alveoli in the lungs open. This method is used for babies who aren't quite getting enough oxygen with the above measures but are still breathing adequately on their own and don't require mechanical ventilation.

Mechanical ventilation. Some babies' lungs are simply too immature (i.e., they don't have enough surfactant for the alveoli to open up) to get enough oxygen using any of the above measures. In this case, the baby is intubated and placed on a ventilator (called a vent) machine. A plastic tube (called an ET tube) is inserted down into baby's trachea (windpipe). The tube is taped securely to baby's face, and another long flexible tube connects it to the ventilator. The "vent" is then set to deliver breaths of air into the baby's lungs at regular intervals. The oxygen concentration in this air can be adjusted to maintain the proper oxygen level in baby's bloodstream. The frequency of breaths and air pressure are adjusted based on the severity of baby's lung problems. Babies with severely immature lungs, who need higher ventilator settings (high pressure, high oxygen concentration, and frequent breaths), may be given sedative medication through an IV so that they sleep while the ventilator does its work. Babies who require only low ventilator settings (low pressure, low oxygen concentration, and less frequent breaths) stay awake and take breaths on their own in between ventilator breaths. You'll notice that the doctor or nurse will frequently adjust the settings on the ventilator to be sure your baby is getting the right amount of oxygen and air according to her changing needs. Sometimes the ventilator does all the breathing work for your baby. Other times it only assists your baby, giving her extra breaths so that she doesn't have to work so hard to breathe. When baby is doing most of her own breathing, you may hear the nurses say that she is "triggering the ventilator on her own."

In certain medical situations, an alternative form of ventilation may be used. One type is called high-frequency ventilation. Instead of delivering deep breaths fifteen to thirty times per minute like a standard vent, this type delivers hundreds of tiny puffs of air each minute.

Another alternative method is called liquid ventilation. Baby is sedated with medications, and an oxygen-rich liquid is pumped through the ventilator tube into the baby's lungs. For the few babies who don't do well on the air ventilators described above, liquid oxygen ventilation is a good alternative.

Ventilator medications. Two medications can be administered during ventilation that may help baby breathe more easily. Surfactant (described on page 33) can be pumped into the lungs to improve lung function until baby begins producing his own surfactant. Nitric oxide is a gas that can be added to the ventilator air to help keep the blood vessels in the lungs open and better able to absorb oxygen. This is used only when baby's very immature lungs need extra support.

Chest X-rays. Virtually all preemies will get at least one X-ray of the chest to assess the status of the lungs. Babies on a ventilator will typically get a chest X-ray every morning to better monitor the condition of the lungs and the position of the ET tube. You need not worry about "all that radiation exposure." Modern X-ray equipment delivers only a tiny amount of radiation, and any risk involved is outweighed by the benefits of having accurate information to use in making decisions about your baby's treatment.

Questions You Might Have About Ventilators

How long will my baby need to be on a ventilator?

If your baby was born extremely premature (prior to 30 weeks), he will probably require a ventilator for a few weeks. If your baby was born at 30 weeks or later, his time on the ventilator may be only a matter of days. Of course, every baby is different, and there is really no way to predict this for sure. If baby is requiring high ventilator settings (high pressure and frequency of breaths and high percentage of oxygen), then it will be a while before baby comes off the ventilator. When baby is breathing some on his own and requiring low ventilator settings,

then he may be close to being weaned off the ventilator.

How is my baby weaned off the ventilator?

Your baby's doctor, nurse, and respiratory therapist will frequently adjust the oxygen and ventilator settings to see how baby tolerates lower settings. They will use blood gas testing (see page 46) and oxygen saturation monitors to determine how your baby is handling the gradually lowered settings. If all is going well, they will continue to decrease the vent settings. Typically, only one or two small weaning steps will be made daily, and there may be days when your baby cannot tolerate lowering the settings. If baby has been sedated because of the high settings on the ventilator, the IV sedation will also be decreased gradually to allow baby to breathe more on his own. Eventually the vent will be set so low and baby will be "breathing around the vent" so well that the breathing tube will be removed (a process called extubation). Of course, baby may continue to need oxygen for varying periods of time through less invasive techniques (see Oxygen, page 33), but eventually he will be weaned from this as well.

NEUROLOGIC SYSTEM

Your baby's developing nervous system is of prime importance to the medical team. There are two primary goals of initial preemie intensive care that are aimed at protecting baby's brain: (1) to maintain adequate oxygen delivery to baby's fragile brain (discussed above); and (2) to ensure adequate blood flow to the brain by maintaining appropriate blood pressure and heart function (discussed below).

The doctors will periodically assess your baby's neurologic health by examining his reflexes, muscle tone, pupils, and the movements of his extremities. Some younger preemies will also have an ultrasound of the brain (called a cranial ultrasound) to check for various problems within the brain (see Intraventricular Hemorrhage, page 202). Rarely, preemies will exhibit seizure symptoms (rapid shaking of the limbs or facial muscles), which can be an indication of neurologic problems (see Seizures, page 207).

During this intensive care, what is your baby feeling? How much is your baby aware of what is going on around her and what is being done to her? Does she feel pain? Is she stressed? These are concerns that your baby's medical team will pay close attention to. There are several ways these issues are cared for during the period of intensive care:

Muscle relaxation. A baby will naturally try to cry and squirm while on a ventilator. Such efforts interfere with the effectiveness of the ventilator breaths and oxygenation. In this situation, baby is given an IV medication that paralyzes the muscles so the relaxed lungs will allow the ventilator to do its job. This effect is temporary and wears off when the medication is stopped and baby is ready for weaning off the ventilator.

Sedation. Some babies don't need full paralysis during intensive care. They may just need some relaxing sedation so they don't waste precious energy from the stress and agitation that intensive care can create.

Pain medications. The various lines, tubes, and procedures used during intensive care can be painful for baby. Pain causes baby to waste valuable energy and calories. IV pain medications are routinely given to keep baby comfortable. For a list of these medications, see Medications Most Commonly Used in the NICU, page 45.

Weaning off medications. As baby's respiratory status improves and he doesn't need as much ventilator support, these medications will be decreased so baby can wake up more, move around, and start breathing on his own. There are no lasting neurologic effects from these medications.

CARDIOVASCULAR SYSTEM

A well-functioning cardiovascular system is required to deliver all this oxygen through the bloodstream to all the parts of baby's body. The cardiovascular system is made up of the heart, which pumps the blood, and the blood vessels through which it travels. In the first hours after birth, some preemies may have problems with inadequate cardiovascular function (low blood pressure and poor blood flow). These problems typically are resolved when the respiratory system is stabilized through the use of oxygen or other assistance with breathing. If the doctors determine that the heart isn't working well despite adequate oxygen and ventilation, the following measures are typically undertaken to improve your baby's blood flow and blood pressure:

• Fluids are given quickly through a large IV, usually the umbilical IV (see Intravenous Lines, below). These fluids expand baby's blood volume, which in turn improves cardiovascular function.

• Blood pressure medications are given through an IV. Those most commonly used are dopamine, dobutamine, and epinephrine. These constrict baby's less important blood vessels, raising the blood pressure and improving blood flow to baby's vital organs. Baby will be weaned off these medications as soon as possible.

If your baby's status isn't improving with these measures, the doctors may need to evaluate baby's heart. An ultrasound of the heart, called an echocardiogram, may be done to check for any heart problems.

Breathing and heart rate leads. Throughout your baby's stay in the NICU, her heart rate will be continuously monitored. It's especially important for the monitor to detect slower than optimal breathing (called apnea) or slower than optimal heart rate (called bradycardia).

You will notice three "leads" — tiny, quarter-size patches, two on her chest and one on her leg or tummy — that are attached to wires that are connected to a monitor. Information about baby's heart and breathing rate is recorded and displayed on a screen. When you look at the monitor, you'll notice that baby's heart beats fast and she breathes much faster than you do. A preemie's heart rate is normally from 120 to 160 beats per minute. Preemie breathing rates typically range from 30 to 60 breaths a minute. The monitor alarm may sound if baby's heart rate and breathing rate stray outside these preset limits. Expect false alarms when these leads are jostled as baby moves. The

nurse will often watch the baby closely instead of the monitor, especially when there is an alarm. You, too, can learn to watch your baby and recognize when her normal skin color and breathing movements do not jibe with the monitor alarms.

Intravenous lines. Called IVs or lines for short, these tiny tubes inserted into a vein provide a route for giving baby fluids, medicines, and nutrients. The opening into baby's vein can also be used to draw blood samples. Sometimes the IV is connected to a continuous infusion pump, which automatically delivers a preset amount of fluid to your baby. Some IVs are capped off with a plastic device called a heparin lock (or Hep-Lock), which prevents the blood from clotting and keeps the vein open. This makes it possible for the doctors and nurses to draw blood or administer medicine without having to repeatedly stick baby with a needle. These IVs may be designated TKO, NICU lingo for "to keep open," just in case they are needed. At times they will be connected to pumps or "drips," so that medication can be administered at a steady rate right into baby's bloodstream. These pumps usually have alarms that sound if the vein or tubing becomes clogged. Ask the nurse to tell you about your baby's IV, why it is there, and what it is being used for. The nurse can also tell you what to do if the alarm goes off or if there seems to be a problem with baby's IV that is not detected by the monitor. Knowing what all the tubing is for and how you can tell if it's working correctly is just another way of keeping connected to and involved with your baby.

Everyone is familiar with the standard IV line that is placed in an adult patient's arm, on the inside of the wrist or elbow. However, when the patient is a newborn baby, IVs are placed in different sites, and different types of intravenous lines are used for different purposes, such as to deliver medicines, fluids, and nutrients. Here are the types of IV that may be used for your baby:

- *Standard peripheral IV.* This type of IV uses a needle to insert a tiny plastic catheter about 1 inch deep into baby's vein. The needle is removed, the catheter remains in baby's vein, and the IV is secured to baby's skin with tape. Usually the IV is placed in baby's forearm, hand, leg, or foot. A large vein on the scalp is another easily accessible site. These IVs typically last for only 1 to 3 days, and then a new one may need to be inserted elsewhere.
- *Percutaneous catheter.* This is a longer-lasting IV that is usually placed in the arm or leg. The tubing extends several inches up the vein to a longer or "central" vein. Tiny stitches are used to secure the line to baby's skin so that it cannot be pulled out accidentally. This type of IV is used when a baby is expected to need IV therapy for a week or more. The main advantage of this "perc line" is that it delivers fluids and medications to larger veins deep in baby's body and is therefore less irritating.
- *Umbilical vein catheter.* When it is apparent that a newborn is going to require serious intensive care, this catheter is painlessly and easily inserted by a doctor several inches into the large vein in baby's umbilical cord stump (still fresh from birth). It is secured with tiny

stitches. This catheter is a convenient place to give IV fluids and medications, as well as draw out blood samples for testing. It can be used for about 1 week.
- *Umbilical artery catheter.* This catheter acts as both a monitor and a conduit for blood test samples. The umbilical artery runs alongside the umbilical vein. This line is not used for giving fluids or medications. Instead, the tubing has sensors at the tip that can measure baby's blood pressure very accurately, which is very useful information if baby's cardiovascular status is unstable. Arterial blood samples can also be drawn to accurately measure baby's oxygen and other blood gas levels (see Blood Tests, page 44). A similar catheter, called an art line, can be placed in an artery in the arm.
- *Central line.* The longest-lasting type of IV is a central line. It is usually placed by a pediatric surgeon in an operating room rather than by a NICU nurse. Occasionally the procedure is done in the NICU by the surgeon or the neonatologist. The central line can be placed in the upper arm, upper chest, or in the groin. A small incision is made in the skin to access the vein. The catheter is inserted several inches so that the tip extends up the large vein almost to the heart itself. A central line is used in preemies who will require many weeks of IV therapy due to severe problems, or in babies with intestinal problems who must get their nutrition through the IV.

If your baby is too immature to receive milk feedings through a nasogastric tube (see page 19), he will receive fluids through his intravenous line to keep him well nourished and hydrated until his intestines are mature enough for milk feedings.

GASTROINTESTINAL SYSTEM

One of the most pressing questions parents of preemies ask is "When can I feed my baby?" This is only natural, because feeding is the single most important thing parents do for babies in the first months of life. Parents of preemies are eager to experience this normal part of parenting their newborn.

Preemies are typically not breastfed or bottlefed until their respiratory and cardiovascular systems are stable. A baby certainly can't feed while on a ventilator. And even a baby who does not require a ventilator may still have significant problems with breathing that would make oral feeding difficult. Coordinating breathing, sucking, and swallowing would use too much energy. Two requirements must be met before baby can begin breast- or bottle-feeding: baby's breathing must be fairly comfortable, and baby must be able to suck and swallow. Prior to 32 to 34 weeks of age, most babies cannot coordinate sucking, swallowing, and breathing well enough to nipple-feed. So how will your baby be fed in the meantime? There are two main ways to provide nutrition to a premature baby: enteral feeding (feeding into the stomach) and parenteral feeding (feeding intravenously).

Enteral feeding. Within a few days of birth, a thin tube is passed through baby's nose or mouth into his stomach. Breast milk or formula is slowly dripped down the tube. This method is also called ga-vage feeding. Many babies are fed continuously in the early weeks. Later, babies get their milk in larger amounts at regular intervals — like they would if they were feeding from a breast or bottle. Premature babies do not have a gag reflex until around 35 weeks, so the feeding tube can usually be left in place without bothering baby. Alternatively, the tube can be inserted and removed with every feeding if baby does seem bothered by it. (See Gavage Feeding, page 126.)

Parenteral feeding. The word "parenteral" doesn't have anything to do with parental, as in Mom and Dad. It literally means feeding "outside of the intestinal system." Why can't a young preemie start enteral feeding right away? Prior to 28 weeks' gestational age, the lining of the intestines is too immature to absorb food well. In fact, food is so irritating to the intestinal lining that it can cause substantial damage and lead to a life-threatening condition called necrotizing enterocolitis (NEC), discussed in detail in chapter 12. So until a baby reaches 28 weeks, she will be fed intravenously.

Intravenous nutrition is called total parenteral nutrition (TPN) or hyperalimentation. You will hear your nurse and doctor use these terms often. The TPN solution contains proteins, fats, sugar, vitamins, and minerals, all in liquid form. It is prepared in an IV bag and given to your baby through an IV.

A typical preemie's nutritional progress will go something like this: Baby is born at 30 weeks' gestation. During the first few days, baby is supported on a ventilator and receives regular IV fluids. Around day

3, baby begins TPN through a perc line, an IV tube placed in his arm (see Percutaneous Catheter, page 38). When baby reaches around 32 weeks of gestational age, the nurses try giving baby some sugar water through a feeding tube. Baby tolerates this well, so he goes on to milk feedings, preferably breast milk pumped by his mother in the first days after the birth and stored in anticipation of this day. Baby tolerates this well, so the volume of TPN he receives is decreased over the next several days and the volume of breast milk, given through the feeding tube as a continuous slow drip, is increased. Baby's intestines handle this transition well and the TPN is stopped. Over the next week, baby's continuous drip feeds are consolidated into intermittent feeds every two to three hours. Once baby reaches the gestational age of 33 or 34 weeks, the nurses and parents begin teaching baby how to nipple-feed, either at the breast or with a bottle. It may take many days for baby to develop a well-coordinated "suck, swallow, and breathing" pattern, but eventually he is able to get all his nutrition from the breast or bottle and he is weaned off the tube feedings. (See The Feeding Sequence, page 122.)

Weight Gain

During the first few days, expect baby to lose rather than gain weight. Both full-term and premature babies are born with extra body fluid that is eliminated through the urine in the first days after birth. Once the respiratory and other systems are stabilized and the day-to-day care becomes more routine, most babies will begin to gain around ½ to 1 ounce (15 to 30 grams) per day. You can plot and track baby's weight gain over the coming weeks on the preemie growth chart on page 219.

The nurses and doctors in the NICU will discuss your baby's weight in grams or kilograms. NICUs use the metric system because all medications and IV fluids are dosed precisely according to baby's weight in kilograms. If you have trouble converting to the metric system, ask a nurse to translate baby's weight into pounds and ounces. You can also use the weight conversion table on page 213 of this book. Most NICUs used to have a certain weight that babies needed to meet before going home (generally around 4¼ pounds or 2200 grams), but many have abandoned this as a necessary criterion for discharge home. The main criterion for your baby's discharge is a demonstrated steady weight gain on breast or bottle feedings without needing tube feedings.

TEMPERATURE REGULATION

Full-term infants are able to maintain a normal body temperature regardless of the temperature in the room. A baby's nervous system detects any changes in body temperature and tells the cardiovascular system to fix the problem. Because this system is immature in preemies, they are not able to keep themselves warm in the open air. This is why your baby is cared for either on a warming table under a heat light or inside a transparent isolette. The thermostat in the isolette is set to maintain a stable, comfortable temperature, normally around 98.6° F (37° C), so that baby stays warm. The digital display on the front reports the isolette's temperature setting and baby's current body temperature (measured by a small sensor taped to baby's abdomen). When baby's body temperature falls too low, the isolette's heater comes on to warm baby up. As baby matures and is able to maintain a stable body temperature by herself, the nurse will open up the front walls of the isolette and turn the heater off. If baby continues to be able to keep herself warm, she will be moved to a regular open crib. This is referred to as weaning to an open crib. This is a fun milestone for parents because now they can enjoy unlimited access to their baby. Most babies are able to regulate their own body temperature when they reach approximately 4 pounds (1800 grams).

INFECTION CONTROL

Although most cases of premature delivery don't have an identifiable cause, a common known cause is infection. There are several different kinds of bacterial infections the mother may carry that can induce premature labor. Your baby will be checked for the presence of such infections, using blood samples and other tests. However, it may take two or more days for the lab to determine if an infection is present and to identify the appropriate antibiotics for the most likely culprit. In the meantime, until the doctors are sure no infection is present, your baby may receive antibiotics through an IV. If an infection is found, your baby may receive antibiotics for around 10 days.

One common source of infection for preemies is the people around them and the medical equipment used to care for them. Bacteria are everywhere. This is why your baby's environment is kept as sterile as possible. But preemies have a very immature immune system, and not only are they susceptible to catching an infection, but germs can easily spread rapidly through baby's system, and an infection can become severe quickly. This is why most doctors are quite aggressive in testing for and treating infections in the NICU. (For more information on infections, see chapter 12.)

ROUTINE NURSING CARE

You will notice that NICU nurses are almost constantly busy doing something. They do far more than just give babies their medicine and help the doctors. Nurses have a number of important tasks they perform at regular intervals, and their observations and test results are recorded in baby's vital sign flow sheet. With this flow sheet, the doctor and other medical personnel can get a quick indication of how baby is doing (besides just looking at your baby.) Flow sheets are either a handwritten record, with a new flow sheet used every day, or a computerized record. Here is a brief explanation of what the nurses do with your baby every day and why.

Perform physical exams. Whereas the doctors examine your baby one or more times each day, the nurses do so more often. This is an important part of closely observing your baby for improvements or problems, and it is more often a nurse than a doctor who will find subtle changes in your baby that require attention.

Check vital signs. The nurses check these at regular intervals and record the results on baby's flow sheet. Some more advanced computers automatically store baby's vital information. More critically ill babies have their vitals checked continuously and recorded every hour. Stable

PREEMIE PAIN

It certainly hurts your heart to see your baby all "wired up and tubed." But how much does this hurt baby? The NICU staff are very mindful that there is a little person on the receiving end of all those needles and tubes, and they try their best to minimize the pain associated with the various procedures. While preemies can't speak, and may not even cry very much, they do feel. When drawing blood or inserting an IV, doctors and nurses watch for changes in baby's vital signs. Studies show that when babies hurt, their breathing rate, heart rate, and blood pressure may rise and the oxygen level in their blood may fall. Babies may also become agitated, stiffen their bodies, arch their backs, jerk, or twitch when they are in pain. Some astute doctors and nurses can pick up on very subtle signs of pain in preemies. With modern NICU treatment, the neonatal staff are able to keep babies even more comfortable. Since pain and stress can slow a preemie's healing and growth, the NICU staff make a special effort to keep your baby as comfortable as possible and minimize the number of needle sticks and other potentially painful procedures.

Learn to watch your baby for signs of discomfort, and speak up for your baby when you think something is bothering her. To relieve the discomfort, your baby may be sedated, especially if there are uncomfortable prongs in her nose or a tube in her trachea (windpipe). Surprisingly, many babies accept these breathing tubes without protest, but some need sedation to keep them calm. Sedation is especially important if baby "fights" the ventilator and therefore is not breathing effectively.

Some medications lessen pain (analgesics), and others calm the upset baby (sedatives). The neonatologist may be reluctant to prescribe an analgesic or sedative for your baby, since these medications may interfere with optimal breathing and heart rate. The doctor has to weigh the risks and benefits of medication when making a decision about what's best for your baby.

Meanwhile, you can try these natural ways to lessen your baby's discomfort. Here's where parents shine:

- Apply skin-to-skin contact. Gently stroke your baby's skin or lay your open hand on his back or abdomen. If baby can be taken out of the isolette, drape him skin-to-skin over your chest. (See Practice Kangaroo Care, page 68.) Babies tolerate painful procedures such as blood drawing better when being held by their parents.
- Give your baby a pacifier dipped in your breast milk or sugar water. Sucking helps to relieve pain.
- Turn down the lights and noise around your baby, and minimize any potentially upsetting stimulation.
- Sing to your baby or play soothing music. Sometimes hand swaddling your baby for a few minutes will help. (See Lay On a Warm Hand, page 60.)

babies might have them checked only every 4 hours.

- *Temperature.* Doctors and nurses like to see baby maintain a stable temperature. The nurse will use the skin sensor already taped to baby's abdomen to check baby's temperature. A rectal or underarm temperature may also be checked occasionally for greater accuracy. If the "temp" is consistently too low, or if baby runs a fever, it could mean he is fighting an infection.
- *Heart rate.* This fluctuates continually minute by minute, so the nurses watch for the overall trend in baby's heart rate. If the heart rate steadily increases over a few hours, say, from 140 beats per minute up to 170, this can mean baby is agitated, dehydrated, anemic, or fighting an infection.
- *Respiratory rate.* Generally, the slower the breathing rate, the more stable is baby's respiratory status. If the breathing rate suddenly or gradually increases, baby's lungs have to work harder to absorb enough oxygen. The nurses and doctors will act promptly to evaluate this.
- *Blood pressure.* This is an accurate measure of how baby's cardiovascular system is working. A drop in blood pressure can indicate a variety of problems, such as infection, shock, or decreased heart function. The cause will be promptly assessed. Some babies experience high blood pressure due to agitation, pain, decreased kidney function, or the overall stress of intensive care.

Measure fluid balance. Maintaining an even fluid balance is critical for young preemies. It's fairly easy to measure every

cc of IV fluid, breast milk, or formula that goes into baby, but it's more challenging to record every cc that comes out. Keeping an accurate record of baby's Is and Os (ins and outs) is a continuous challenge for nurses. Here is what they measure and how they do it:

- *Urine output.* Critically ill young preemies have their urine continuously collected by a catheter inserted into the bladder. This amount is measured throughout the day. As baby stabilizes, she simply pees into a diaper. The diapers are weighed to determine how much urine is there.
- *Urine dipstick test.* This test is done several times each day to monitor baby's urine for sugar, blood, protein, and specific gravity. The "spec grav" is an indication of how hydrated a baby is. If the nurse notices a consistently high spec grav, it may mean baby is getting dehydrated.
- *Stool output.* Nurses monitor baby's stools to help keep track of baby's output.
- *Stool heme or guiac test.* This test checks for blood in baby's stools. Nurses do this at least once a day.
- *Intake.* Nurses write down the hourly amount of IV fluid and oral feeds that baby gets. The required amount is carefully calculated by the doctor based on baby's weight and age.
- *Incidental losses.* Baby loses some body fluids from evaporation through the skin and from breathing. This is taken into consideration when determining baby's fluid balance.

Every 12 hours, or more frequently in the case of sicker preemies, the nurses add up baby's total intake and output. Typically, baby will take in slightly more than she puts out. If input far exceeds output, baby will become swollen, which puts a strain on all of her body organs. If the output is greater than what baby takes in, she may become dehydrated. The nurses and doctors will adjust baby's intake to keep things in balance.

Check weight. Baby's weight is checked once or twice a day. While baby is expected to slowly gain weight, too much weight gain in a single day or two can mean baby's intake is too great.

Monitor the monitors. The nurses periodically check all of baby's IVs and monitor wires to make sure everything is functioning properly.

Administer heel stick blood tests. While the laboratory does more complex blood testing, the nurses may perform a couple of simple tests on a few drops of blood from baby's heel:

- *Blood sugar.* It is important to check this once or twice a day in more critical young preemies, as they are prone to sudden low or high blood sugar fluctuations.
- *Hematocrit.* This simple test for anemia can be done at the bedside in some NICUs.

BLOOD TESTS

There may be times during your baby's stay in the NICU when you worry about "all those pokes." In the early critical days of baby's care, blood samples may be drawn several times a day. As baby stabilizes, the need for blood testing dimin-ishes. Doctors and nurses try their best to order only those tests that are necessary. If your baby has a central line or umbilical vein catheter, obtaining blood samples is easy and painless. However, not all babies have IVs that provide such easy access, and it's difficult for a parent to watch a nurse or technician use a needle to draw blood from baby's arm day in and day out.

These are the most common blood tests that you may hear the staff discuss:

CBC. This complete blood count measures the concentration of various types of blood cells, including the following:

- *White blood cells.* If these levels are high or extremely low, your baby may be fighting an infection.
- *Hemoglobin or hematocrit.* This is a measure of the red blood cell concentration. If it is low, baby is anemic. See page 189 for a full discussion of anemia.
- *Platelets.* These tiny cells help blood form clots to stop bleeding. Occasionally the level will be low enough that a platelet transfusion will be needed.

Basic metabolic panel. This test measures levels of various important minerals, as well as blood sugar and kidney function.

Comprehensive metabolic panel. This test measures the same levels and functions as the basic metabolic panel, and also assesses the health of various organ systems.

Bilirubin. Bilirubin is a yellow pigment that builds up in baby's skin during the first few days of life. It will be measured if your baby's skin begins to appear yellow or jaundiced. See page 193 for a full discussion of jaundice.

Blood cultures. The lab uses a blood sample to determine if there is a bacterial infection in baby's bloodstream.

Blood sugar level. During critical phases in baby's care, this may be measured more than once a day. You may hear it

---

MEDICATIONS MOST COMMONLY USED IN THE NICU

You will hear the medical staff discussing the various medications your baby is being given. You will also see IV medications attached to baby's IV pump or written on the nursing flow sheet. It's challenging for a parent to remember what each medicine does and why it is being given. Here is a quick-reference guide that you can use to keep it all clear in your mind.

Antibiotics. The most commonly used are ampicillin, gentamycin, vancomycin, and cefotaxime. Two antibiotics are often used together for better treatment and are given intravenously.

Antacids. Zantac and cimetidine are the most common. They are used while baby is getting TPN (IV nutrition) to decrease the stomach acid, which can be irritating to baby's empty stomach. They are also used for babies with gastroesophageal reflux (see page 195).

Reglan. This medication is used for some babies with gastroesophageal reflux (see page 195) to help food move through the stomach faster.

Steroids. These are occasionally used when baby is critically ill or extremely stressed. Used appropriately, steroids are very safe and their benefits far outweigh any risks.

Diuretics. Lasix and Diuril are most commonly used. These increase urine production so that babies who have taken in too much fluid can eliminate excess fluids.

Muscle relaxants. Atracurium, pancuronium, and vecuronium are common muscle relaxants. These are used in very premature babies to keep their muscles completely relaxed so the ventilator can effectively breathe for baby. (See Neurologic System, page 35.)

Pain medications. Fentanyl is commonly used to ease the discomfort of invasive intensive care and allow baby to rest and conserve energy.

Sedatives. Versed and Ativan are common sedatives. They relax baby during invasive intensive care and painful procedures.

Cardiac medications. Dopamine and dobutamine are commonly used to raise baby's blood pressure when baby's heart is not functioning adequately. (See Cardiovascular System, page 36.)

Apnea medications. Aminophylline is an IV medication used to prevent apnea spells. (See Apnea of Prematurity, page 191.) Theophylline and caffeine are similar and given by mouth.

referred to as a chem strip or Accu-Chek test. Very high or very low sugar levels can cause baby's blood to be out of biochemical balance.

Blood gases. This test measures the levels of oxygen, carbon dioxide, and acid in baby's blood. These all need to be in proper balance in order for baby to grow. If baby is on a ventilator, this test is performed one or more times daily to monitor how baby is doing. Blood samples can be taken from an arterial catheter (referred to as arterial blood gas, or ABG), a vein or IV catheter (termed a venous blood gas, or VBG), or from the capillaries in the heel, using a pin prick (termed a capillary blood gas, or cap gas).

For more information about medical tests, see the glossary on page 229.

TESTS AND PROCEDURES MOST COMMONLY DONE IN THE NICU

It helps to be familiar with some of the major tests and procedures that may be performed to monitor your baby's progress and evaluate any complications:

Cranial ultrasound. Just like the ultrasound you had during pregnancy, this is a painless and noninvasive test. The ultrasound probe is placed on baby's soft spot on top of the skull to obtain images of the brain. It is done to check for bleeding or swelling in the brain (see Intraventricular Hemorrhage, page 202, and Hydrocephalus, page 203). It is not done on all babies.

X-rays. Typically, preemies will get several X-rays of their chest and abdomen. Each X-ray is only a tiny amount of radiation, and there are no immediate or long-term effects from such minute exposures.

Lumbar puncture (spinal tap). This test is done in order to determine if baby has meningitis. It is not done on all babies.

Echocardiogram (ECHO). This is an ultrasound of the heart. It is painless and noninvasive and is done to check for heart defects and to assess heart function. It is not done on all babies.

Electrocardiogram (EKG). In this test, monitor wires are taped to baby's chest, and the electrical activity of the heart is measured to assess heart function. It is painless and noninvasive.

Electroencephalogram (EEG). To evaluate baby for seizures, monitor wires are taped to baby's head, and the electrical activity of the brain is measured. It is not done on all babies.

Pneumogram, or sleep study. This noninvasive and painless test is done to evaluate baby for Apnea spells (see page 191). During sleep, baby's heart rate, breathing, and blood oxygen concentration are continuously measured.

If your doctor or nurse tells you about a potential problem, such as a high bilirubin level, don't panic. Get informed. Ask questions: What does this mean? Is it serious? What are the potential problems? Get all

the information before you fret. Once I learned that a high bilirubin level was usual in preemies, I didn't worry as much. I wish they had told me that in the first place.

Congratulations! You have completed Neonatology 101. You are well on your way to a basic understanding of your baby's medical care. In chapter 12, we will go into more detail about the most common medical challenges your baby may face. Now that you have a deeper understanding of what your preemie needs — and now that you are better prepared to help — read on.

DONATE YOUR BLOOD FOR BABY

At some point your baby may need a blood transfusion. See page 190 to read about how to donate your blood early so it will be ready for baby if needed.

Working Through Your Fears and Feelings

PARENTS OF PREEMIES spend the first weeks or months of baby's life on emotional overload. Life is not turning out as planned, and you're left feeling angry, scared, and lonely. Having a baby was supposed to be a joyful event. How are you supposed to cope when you can't even hold your baby in your arms?

The previous chapters in this book had a lot to say about your baby's health and the technology that is used to help your baby grow and thrive until he is ready to go home. We feel that it's helpful for you to know all this, but we also understand that right now, nothing is as real to you as the emotions spinning around inside you. These feelings are important. How you resolve them will affect how you feel about your role as a parent. Identifying these feelings and talking about them are the first steps toward resolving them. This chapter describes the feelings that parents — especially mothers — who have had a premature baby had and the way they coped with those feelings.

We are richer as human beings for having had the privilege of parenting a preemie.

Robbed. You were expecting a mostly blissful nine-month pregnancy and a full-term healthy baby. But this is not what you got. Your response: "I've been robbed! I deserved better!"

Well-meaning but clueless friends or relatives may try to comfort you: "But the doctors say your baby is going to be okay. Be glad." But you're not glad. You feel as if you've been cheated out of those early moments, days, and weeks of motherhood. You may not even have been able to complete your childbirth or parenting classes. You're lying in a hospital bed while your baby lies in a plastic box on another floor, or even in another hospital. You may mourn the loss of the rest of your pregnancy and resent being robbed of those extra weeks you needed to get ready to be a mom. Perhaps you had to leave your job sooner than expected and didn't have time to prepare for your departure. Perhaps the nursery isn't finished. Meanwhile, other mothers get to nurse and caress their babies. Why not you?

It's natural to feel this way when pregnancy ends too early. Some mothers of preemies even feel "incomplete" as mothers because they were not able to carry their baby to term. It's important to acknowledge to yourself that you have experienced real, legitimate losses — even if your baby's prognosis is good. It's natural to grieve over the pregnancy and birth experience you lost.

The first day I felt cheated because I couldn't hold him, room-in with him, and breastfeed right away.

Unnatural. What could be more unnatural than life in the NICU? You may feel like you're living in a science-fiction movie. It's unnatural for mother and baby to be separated at birth, unnatural to view your baby through a plastic box, unnatural to see him fed through a tube and to have to imagine what he looks and feels like under all those patches and tubes. Nature provides ways for parents to fall in love with their babies, such as skin contact, eye-to-eye gazing, breastfeeding, and holding. It feels wrong when you don't get to do these things. It's very unnatural not to be able to touch and hold your own child when your whole being — body, mind, and soul — is aching to do so. Caring for your baby at arm's length through plastic portholes does not satisfy this natural craving.

The pain of having to leave her when it was time to go was terrible. I wanted so much to tuck her inside my coat and take her with me!

◆

Every day I struggled as I had to ask permission to touch, hold, and feed my own baby!

◆

The absolute hardest thing that I have ever done and the worst day of my life was when I was discharged from the hospital without my baby. I sat in the lobby waiting for the car and watched other families leaving in celebration with little ones in tow. It was horribly painful, and the feeling will stay with me forever. It's just unnatural to leave the hospital without your baby. Every time I leave the NICU without my baby, it's like a rerun of the pain of that first day.

Overwhelmed. The neonatologist and NICU nurse will come to speak to you right away after your baby is born. Other medical personnel may be hovering around you, too. You're suddenly deluged with forms to sign (and understand!), instructions to comprehend, NICU policies to remember, and complicated explanations of the care being given to your baby. You go to visit your baby in the NICU, and the experience — all those machines, all those tiny babies! — is overwhelming. You're trying to cope with the shock of your baby's early birth and your fears of what lies ahead for your family. You're not sure whether to stay with your baby or run away and sleep.

Dr. Jim advises: Oftentimes you may not want to be "part of the medical team" and learn about all this high-tech stuff. You just want to be a mother. Good! That's just what your baby needs you to be.

The NICU staff was very confident, but there's a sense that they see this every day and it's all "routine" to them. Sometimes they do not appreciate how far behind the parents can be in trying to understand, appreciate, and cope with all that is going on, let alone assimilate all of the medical and technical information they are spewing at you while you are just standing there wondering why you aren't still pregnant!

◆

I felt like I was experiencing a sort of posttraumatic stress disorder.

◆

I felt a combination of anxiety and denial. She was so sick in the beginning that we just operated on autopilot and tried to make it through the day.

Dr. Bill advises: During those first few days, when you're overwhelmed and in a state of shock, don't expect to comprehend everything all at once. NICU staff members know that parents are living in a fog during these first days. They have talked with many parents of preemies, and some of them may even have had premature babies themselves. No one expects you to be perfect or patient, or to comprehend everything you're told. At best, 25 percent of what you hear will sink in the first time. If you don't understand something the first time, ask the doctor or nurse to repeat the information. The NICU staff is used to repeating things many times. Yet, different people have different personalities, and everyone on the NICU staff is only human. Some are more patient than others. Seek out these individuals when you're feeling especially anxious, and be patient with the others. If the doctor isn't immediately available, consult this book.

On an emotional roller coaster. Your preemie's path to maturity will probably follow a pattern of two steps forward and one step backward. You may leave the NICU in the evening pleased with the progress your baby made that day, only to return the next morning and be greeted with "we had a little setback during the night." Baby was off the ventilator, but now he is back on the breathing machine. You felt optimistic yesterday; today you're discouraged. At your low point, it's hard to believe that you will ever feel better again.

One way to cope is to step back from time to time and take the long view. Your baby's day-to-day progress will have its ups and downs, but if you compare this week with last week, or today with a day two weeks ago, you will probably see an upward trend. Keep a daily journal in which you record information about your baby's progress as well as your own feelings. Take time every week to go back through the pages and read old entries. You will get a feeling for how far you've come. More significant, your child may want to read this diary when she is older. Address some of your feelings as if you are talking to your baby. Let her know how much you love and care for her. Share your feelings honestly. This can be an intimate and special gift to give your child when she grows up.

Oh, that infamous NICU roller coaster. One day we were overjoyed to learn he had gained a few ounces, only to be shell-shocked when we arrived the next day to learn he had not only lost weight but was back on gavage feedings.

Ambivalent. Be prepared for mixed feelings. Ambivalence may strike every morning when you open your eyes. You want to hurry to the NICU to see your baby, but you worry that the day may bring a new crisis. You want to spend every minute you can with your baby, yet you desperately need time for yourself. You want to take your baby home, but you're scared that you won't be able to care for her as well as the nurses do.

Ambivalent feelings may show up when you have to make even simple decisions. Moms who are ready to be discharged from the hospital after the birth may find excuses to stay, rather than go home with empty arms. Do you take the time you need to rest and recover from a cesarean, or do you keep vigil at your baby's crib? You never asked to be in this stressful situation, so it's understandable that part of you wants to avoid it. Acknowledging this to yourself will make it easier to do the things you have to do but may not want to do with your whole heart.

On the one hand, I looked forward to getting my first-morning report on how his night was as soon as I arrived at the NICU. On the other hand, I feared getting the worst: that he had gone backward.

Not close to your baby. Mothers of preemies sometimes confide that they don't feel as if they love their babies. Some have not experienced the rush of warm feelings that they expected would come with motherhood. Sometimes parents feel guilty about this or bewildered.

Don't worry if feelings of love and closeness are slow to develop. Even mothers of healthy, full-term infants may not experience a flood of maternal feelings in the early postpartum period. It takes time for love to grow, and it takes even more

time when you are grieving for the healthy baby you imagined.

When baby is critically ill or very premature, one or both parents may subconsciously "prepare" for the possibility that their baby may not survive. Something inside reasons, "If I don't get too close to my baby, I won't hurt so much if he is taken away from me." They may even delay giving their baby a name and find ways to avoid getting involved with their baby's early care. Keeping some distance between themselves and their baby is a protective mechanism that some parents may use to guard against potential hurt. These feelings are one way of coping with the possibility of loss, though the sadness is unavoidable. On the other hand, some parents feel that they will be better able to cope with their infant's death if they have made every effort to fill his short life with their love.

You may not fall head over heels in love with your baby right from the start, but eventually you will click into "bonding mode." The NICU staff members are used to helping parents with these feelings, so don't be afraid to talk with them. One of the best remedies for not feeling close to your baby is . . . your baby! You don't have to feel warm and loving to stroke her skin or talk softly to her. But if you do these things daily, bonding will follow.

Another bonding-related concern is that your baby won't know that you're her mother (or father). Don't worry about this. She will know how special you are. Your baby has already gotten to know you while in the womb. Even preemies can learn to recognize their mother's and father's voices. In no time, baby will know your special voice, your special touch, and eventually mother's special milk. Even though your baby will have multiple care-givers while in the NICU, there will never be any doubt in your baby's mind about who her parents are.

I shied away from my baby in the first few days, but then the nurses practically forced me to bond with him. I'm now glad they did.

Dr. Bob advises: Bonding is a process, not a one-time postpar-tum event. Missing out on those first few hours and days of parent-infant togetherness will not permanently affect your relationship with your child. Your bond with your child is built of many, many interactions, in babyhood and be-yond. Don't fret about what you missed — work on getting attached to your child right now. The earlier you start, the easier it will be. Bonding with your baby in the NICU will be good for both of you.

Hating waiting. Life in the NICU is one long waiting game. Those first few hours — or more — between delivery and first touching your baby may seem like an eternity. Then you wait for the first chance to hold your baby in your arms, the first feeding, the day you can finally take your precious baby home. And every period of waiting is prolonged by setbacks: "You'll have to wait another day before he's ready to be taken out of the isolette be-cause . . ." "You'll have to postpone going home another day because . . ." Progress seems to come so s-l-o-w-l-y. Weight gain is measured in itty-bitty grams. It's easier to endure the waiting game if you keep your hopes high, without creating dead-lines or timetables. Trying to live one day

at a time is not easy, but looking too far into the future will only make you more impatient.

Our NICU stay was the longest five weeks of my life. Time seemed to stand still.

◆

I hated the word "wait." I always had to wait for some test to be done, or wait until after a feeding, or wait for something else before I could hold him. Finally, I found a way to be involved in all his procedures and feedings, and then I felt less like a pinch hitter and more like a teammate.

Doing double duty. Many parents find they are trying to maintain two "homes." Their time is divided between their home in the NICU and their own home. And then there's all the time spent in the car, driving to and from the hospital. If there are other small children in the family who need regular attention from Mom and Dad, parents feel even more torn. Add to this the possibility that Dad or even Mom may have to return to work before baby is ready to come home, and it's no won-der parents feel they are doing double, even triple, duty. Getting extended family involved can make a big difference in your life.

My mom became the temporary "mother" for my two older kids so I could focus enough energy on my baby. This help was priceless!

Separation anxiety. Separation anxiety usually refers to infants' worries about where Mommy is when they can't see her. When parenting a premature baby, the roles are reversed. You worry about your baby when you are not with him.

When I was away from her, just thinking that no one had time to spend quality touch time with her broke my heart.

Stranger anxiety. Your baby, who came from your body, is suddenly being cared for by a whole parade of strangers. They get to touch your baby, feed your baby, and do all the things you should be doing. Your parenting instincts tell you to protect your baby from these strangers, yet all the doctors and nurses seem to know better than you do what your baby needs. You're a raw recruit, in unfamiliar and scary territory, while they are the veterans. It may be tough to take, but you have to trust them with your baby. Take comfort knowing that they are highly skilled professionals and your baby is getting the best possible care — even if it is from "strangers."

I was afraid that she wouldn't know me as her mom.

Bedside boredom. There may be days when you sit and stare for hours at your baby in the isolette, longing to "do something" for him, but with nothing much you can do. Try to stay busy. Keep a journal, make a scrapbook, read a book (this book!). Socialize. Get to know the other NICU parents. If you knit or sew, make a special handmade present for your baby.

It was frightening to see his little chest go in and out as he struggled for each breath. He looked very scared and was tiny and weak. He was also very restless. But when he tried to pull out his tubes, I knew it meant he had a fighting spirit, and I believed that he was going to be okay.

Helpless. It's normal to feel helpless, even useless. You're overwhelmed by the com-

plexity of all the high-tech equipment and frightened by the "fragility" of your baby. You're afraid to hold her because she's so tiny. Yet, you're afraid not to hold her because you know touch is good for her.

I was at her bedside a lot. But when I was there, I felt like I was in the way and I didn't know what to do. So I figured I better make myself useful. Once I learned how to help and which procedures did what and why they were necessary, I felt less in the way.

◆

My greatest fear was that he was suffering and I was unable to do anything about it.

◆

I didn't know what questions to ask. It took me about two weeks of reading her chart and staring at her hour after hour to understand the workings of the NICU and therefore know how to ask the right questions.

Many new parents feel afraid to ask questions of the NICU staff. They may not want to look "dumb," or they are afraid that their concerns may seem trivial. Remember that the doctors caring for your baby have gone to school for about thirteen years in order to master the intricacies of neonatal medicine. The nurses have at least five years of professional schooling, plus lots of on-the-job training. They don't expect you to know as much as they do. Don't be afraid to ask for simple explanations. When your peace of mind depends on getting an answer, there's no such thing as a "dumb question."

Dr. Bill advises. Don't dwell on what you can't do. Focus on what you *can* do — especially those things that nobody else can do — such as pumping and storing your milk, enjoying skin-to-skin contact with your baby, stroking him, reading up on all the special things you and Dad can do for baby. The best way to overcome the helpless feeling you have when entering unfamiliar territory is to get familiar with it as quickly as you can. You don't have to master every complex detail of your baby's medical chart. Every parent's comfort level is different. In our NICU experience, we have noticed that the more quickly parents become involved in the care of their preemie, the better they cope and the better baby grows.

I didn't get to see my twins because they were whisked away to the NICU. All I wanted to do was be with them, touch them, and hold them. I was so worried about them being suddenly yanked out of my body and taken away to the brightly lit room, getting stuck with needles, hooked up to noisy machines with blinking lights, and being left alone in an isolette. What a way to come into the world. I felt so far away from them and just wanted to hold them and protect them.

◆

When he preferred my breast to the bottle, that really boosted my suffering psyche.

◆

I didn't appreciate the doctors who would come by her incubator but not say anything to me. I really appreciated the ones who did, because it made me feel that they realized I was her parent. I was hurting and needed to feel part of the medical team.

◆

I was not encouraged to read her chart, though a friend of mine who had had a preemie told me that I could. I felt very left out of decisions.

You may find yourself undergoing — or needing to undergo — a personality change as you "study" for your degree in NICU mothering. Perhaps you were once a nice, quiet, somewhat reserved person who was content to let other people make waves. Now you're forced to be assertive, to ask questions, dig more deeply, and require better answers. You may even have to challenge authority — tactfully, of course, but firmly. Expect to feel a bit anxious as you're going through this personality transformation. The staff will be patient. They've seen this happen with parents before. (And you're unlikely to confront them with anything they haven't heard before.) One sure way to play a valuable role in baby's medical team is to provide kangaroo care. This is something only *you* can do. See page 68 to learn how.

Guilty. After delivering a preemie, many mothers feel guilty and are unable to deliver themselves of this guilt. It's common for mothers to blame themselves and their bodies for not carrying a baby to term. Then comes the guilt of not being able to be a supermom to your preemie. You may feel guilty for not being able to pump as much milk as your baby needs. Or you feel guilty for not being by your baby's side twenty-four hours a day. You feel guilty because you are spending too much time in the NICU, depriving your other children of their mom at home. When you're at home, you feel guilty that you're not at the NICU. One moment you feel that you're not doing enough for your baby. The next, you feel that somehow you are asking too much of your baby —

you're overstimulating him or, by trying to feed him at your breast, making things too stressful for him. The guilt doesn't end when you both leave the hospital, especially if your baby continues to have special needs that require ongoing care.

Guilty feelings can spiral out of control. Beating up on yourself won't help you be a better parent. Besides, many of the things you feel guilty about are completely beyond your control. If you could have prevented your baby's premature birth, you would have. If you could be in two places at once, you would be. But you can't be at home and at the hospital at the same time. Even the most sensitive and caring of mothers can't always tell how much stimulation is good for baby. You're learning, too. Sometimes feeling guilty is a way to trick ourselves into believing that we have more control over our lives than we do. But it may be less stressful in the long run to simply accept the fact that life hands us plenty of crummy circumstances that can't be changed. Concentrate on doing what you can for your baby, and let go of the rest. If you want to pump more milk, follow some of the suggestions in this book. If they work, great! If your milk supply is still low, try something else. Or ease up on yourself. Change the things you can change, and let the rest be.

Initially, I blamed my body for what his little body was going through. Later I learned to focus more on what my body could do to help him get through it.

Afraid. There are several stages of fear that come with being the parent of a premature baby. The first fear is often, "Will my baby live?" After you're certain that your baby will survive, you face the fear that she may have developmental problems later on. There are other fears as well, such as the fear that you may not be able to make enough milk and the fear that you might hurt your tiny baby by holding her. As one crisis subsides, you begin to fear the next one. Yet, as your baby grows and gets healthier, you will have more good days than bad and your fears will lessen. Learning more about what you're afraid of is a good strategy for dealing with your fear. The good news is that with modern NICU care, not only do even the tiniest preemies usually survive, but most grow up to be just fine. While many do continue to need extra medical attention, you'll discover that there are many helpful resources available to you and your baby.

My greatest fears were that my daughter wouldn't come home and, if she did, that she would have serious difficulties.

◆

It helps to talk to the veterans. Misery needs some company.

Prone to meltdowns. Nearly every parent of a preemie "loses it" at some time during the NICU journey. There are multiple stresses. Baby is born before her time — stress #1. Baby spends a lot of time in the NICU — stress #2. And parents have to cope with all this during the postpartum period, when moms are tired, their bodies are recovering from labor or a C-section, and their hormones are fluctuating wildly. Fathers are discovering that the carefree couple life they once knew is gone forever, but the bills that are starting to arrive won't go away nearly so easily. Whether you explode in anger or in tears (or both at the same time), meltdowns are completely understandable.

Being constantly on edge, with emotions threatening to erupt like a volcano at any moment, may be a sign that you need to start taking better care of yourself. When you're hungry, tired, or lonely, you are more likely to have a meltdown. When the tape that's running in your head is constantly rehearsing the story of everything that has gone wrong, it won't take more than a few words from a busy, distracted nurse to send you off into the adult version of a toddler tantrum. Get some rest, take a shower, eat well, call a friend, or just sit quietly and meditate. Think about something other than your baby for a change. Take a break from your worries — they'll still be there when you get back.

The stress was coming out as I caught myself biting my lip and pulling my hair. I wanted to scream. The frustration that built up during the months of her hospitalization, when I had to divide my life between home and hospital, was obvious. I begged the doctors, "Please, just let us go home." "One more week," they said. Again I went home in tears.

◆

The doctors were very patient with me, as I had a couple of meltdowns and plentiful tears. I just felt so disappointed that I couldn't take my baby home yet, and my greatest fear was that he wouldn't bond with me because we missed something early on — but of course he did.

Depressed. Some degree of postpartum sadness, or even depression, occurs in many women who deliver term babies, and those rates double for mothers of preemies. Considering that "multiple stresses" are one of the prime triggers for all kinds of depression, it's no wonder that nearly all mothers of preemies experience some degree of postpartum depression in the early weeks and months. Take all your anger, grief, fear, loss of sleep, and separation anxiety from being away from your baby, put them all together, and you have a recipe for depression.

The best help you can give your baby is to take good care of yourself. If you find yourself slipping into a depressed mood that just won't go away, or if your feelings of sadness are hampering your ability to care for and enjoy your baby, seek professional help. The NICU staff will be able to refer you to professional counselors who are experienced in dealing with postpartum depression, which is a very common and treatable problem. You owe it to yourself to get help for your depression as soon as possible.

The nurses became so used to seeing me cry, they kept a box of Kleenex just for me on top of the isolette.

Dreaming about D-day. You'll probably find yourself longing for and imagining departure day, the day you'll *finally* be able to take your baby home. Yet, doctors can only guess at when that day will be. If they are reluctant to be specific, it's because they do not want to disappoint you if they have to rethink their early calculations. Day by day they will watch your baby's progress and tell you what signposts and red flags they are looking for. Wait and watch with them. Chapter 9, Homecoming, will help get you and baby ready for D-day.

I had the privilege of watching my baby grow in the "outside womb" for the last four weeks.

Helping Your Baby Grow in the Hospital

YOUR BABY'S TEAM OF doctors, nurses, and other support staff brings a vast amount of knowledge and experience to the job of providing medical care for your baby. You may think that there is little you can do to add to their efforts. Yet you have something to offer that is equally important to your baby's well-being. You have a genetic, instinctive, emotional connection to your baby that no one else can match. And your baby has this same connection to you. You may not have years of medical training, but you are your baby's parents. No one else can give the emotional and physical comfort that you can. No one else can offer the same kind of support or the same kind of loving care.

Your premature baby needs two kinds of care: medical care to support his physical needs, and touch and affection to support his emotional needs. In this chapter we will show you how research has demonstrated that preemies who receive lots of loving touch grow better and have fewer medical problems. What better preventive medicine could there be? In reality, baby's need for physical touch *is* a

medical need. We will show you ways in which you can involve yourself in baby's care throughout her NICU stay. Your physical care for your baby will not only help her thrive, but it will also help you develop as a parent.

BE YOUR BEST AT BABY'S BEDSIDE

During the time that your baby is in the NICU, you will want to spend as many hours there as possible. Yet you can do much more with this time than sit and stare or just hold baby's tiny hand. Here's how to make the most of your days in the NICU.

Be observant. Watch the doctors, nurses, and other persons who tend to your baby. Read their name tags. Get to know what they do and why. Figure out who reports to whom. Watch the various monitors and machines. After you've observed your surroundings for a while, you will be able to ask the questions that will get you the answers you need.

Above all, observe your baby. Notice her color, her breathing pattern, her facial expressions. Discover your baby's personal quirks. Twitches of the facial muscles or of the arms and legs are a reflection of the immaturity of her nervous system. Baby may even surprise you by sucking her thumb. Observe your baby's signs of discomfort. These are very subtle in preemies and tough to decode — perhaps a facial grimace or a jerky movement. Some may be nothing more than normal preemie immaturity, while others indicate that baby needs soothing. If your baby calms down in response to your loving touch, you'll know that you have made the right call. If a gentle hand on baby's back doesn't seem to help, it may be that baby's movements are nothing more than reflexes at work.

Be involved. After observing what is being done and learning why, ask the nurses how you can help. Certainly you can assist in caring for your baby's personal needs, changing his diapers, bathing him, and perhaps performing some simple procedures, such as chest physiotherapy (gentle tapping on baby's chest to help clear mucus). Ask the nurses to share their observations about your baby with you, to tell you about his color or the changes in

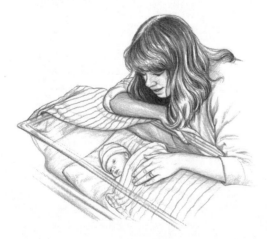

STRESS SIGNS

Just as you notice the body language that tells you baby feels content, notice also her unique, individual signals of stress. Here are some general guidelines to help you tell the difference between contentment and stress.

Signs of contentment:

- Baby's face looks relaxed.
- Baby's limbs are quiet or moving slowly.
- Baby's hands are partially open and fingers are relaxed.

Signs of stress:

- Baby clenches her fists.
- Baby's arms and legs flail around in jerky movements.
- Baby frowns or grimaces.
- Baby's neck and back are arched and her face looks pained.

---

his breathing patterns. This will make you a better baby observer. Ask what all the numbers and squiggly lines on the monitors mean, and use your growing powers of observation to distinguish between false and true alarms. You don't need to keep your eyes nervously fixed on your baby and the monitors. Actually, the more you know about what to look for in your baby, the less you will be bothered by the machinery.

Dr. Jim advises: Keep a watchful eye on your baby. You, the person who was connected to the other end of baby's umbilical cord, may observe things that nobody else will see. Nurses come and go, but parents are forever. You are your baby's one consistent caregiver. Your observations really do matter. You may notice something done by a nurse on a previous shift that made your baby more comfortable. Share this information with the nurse on the next shift ("When we turned him on his left side, the nurse and I noticed that he seemed to breathe better").

Be comfortable. Develop your own "nurse's station" next to baby's bedside. You may need to bring your own rocking chair and pillow, or other comfortable chair. Bring a cooler with drinks and healthy snacks. (You may have to keep these in a room outside the NICU, if that is the unit's policy.) You may also want to bring a personal CD or tape player, with music that is soothing to you. Pack a bag of other things from home that help you feel good, such as unscented hand lotion, a journal or sketchbook, books or magazines, a small photo album, Post-it notes (for leaving notes on baby's isolette), a cheerful picture or greeting card, and a list of phone numbers you may need.

I made a tape of me singing the same songs I sang to her while she was in the womb.

Administer "touch therapy." The best thing you can do at your baby's bedside is caress and touch her (when baby is old enough). Babies who are caressed have fewer episodes of apnea, gain weight faster, and leave the hospital sooner. Your careful observations will help you determine what kind of touching is most soothing for baby. Too much stroking may

irritate very premature babies who may calm better with a steady-pressure type of touch.

LEARN STAGE-APPROPRIATE STIMULATION

Preemies develop differently from term babies. Your baby's behavior, responsiveness, movements, social abilities, and cries will all change as he grows. It's important for you to be aware of your baby's stage of development so that you can better respond to his unique needs. Very tiny preemies will not tolerate much, if any, stimulation. Older preemies crave gentle touching. The following section is an introduction to preemie development and behavior, divided into several age categories. We hope that this information will equip you to respond to your baby in ways appropriate to his age and stage and thus provide the best emotional and physical support you can.

Micropreemies

Babies born at less than 26 weeks' gestation have extremely immature nervous systems and probably won't show much response to stimulation. Yet, after a week or two, you may start to see small movements of the arms and legs, occasional sucking reflexes, and spontaneous breaths. Even though micropreemies show little outward response to stimulation, internally they may respond negatively.

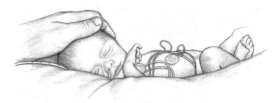

Their heart rate, blood pressure, oxygen levels, and temperature may fluctuate (an indication of stress) when they are moved, touched, or overstimulated in any way.

For this reason, parents are usually not encouraged to touch or stimulate their micropreemie until the body systems are more stable. Take heart. Even though you cannot be physically involved with the baby, by staying close to her bedside, you are nurturing your own attachment to her. Soon you will be able to take a more active part in baby's care.

Extremely Premature Babies

Babies born between 26 and 29 weeks show more spontaneous movements and reactions to stimuli. They spend most of their time sleeping but do wake up briefly and even open their eyes, although not long enough for any prolonged interaction with you. They can see dark-and-light contrasts but cannot focus very well beyond a few inches. Your baby may be able to notice the outline of your head and know you're there, but he cannot distinguish your facial features. Extremely premature babies can hear, but they seldom show any response to sounds and don't even startle at loud noises. Their sense of smell is not yet well developed either. An extremely premature baby will not cry, but you will see signs of distress or excitement, such as changes in body posture, color, and breathing or heart rate, hiccupping, arching of the back, and erratic limb movements. Occasionally, these preemies move spontaneously and stretch, open and close their fists, or even suck on their fingers.

At this early age, your doctors will continue to caution you about overstimulating

baby. Your physical contact with baby may still have to be minimal, depending on how stable your baby is. As you begin to touch your baby, you and your nurse will need to observe baby's vital signs and physical reactions to make sure baby is tolerating this new level of stimulation without stress. Every baby has a unique personality and will respond differently to parents' touch. Here are some ways you can gently stimulate and begin to connect with your baby through physical contact:

Lend a finger. Gently place your fingers in baby's palm and feel your little one's grasp for the first time. This soft grasp is a reflex, not a purposeful movement, but nonetheless it feels very special to parents.

Lay on a warm hand. With baby lying on his tummy, place your relaxed hand over baby's head and back. This is called hand swaddling. (Do not rub or massage — this may be too stimulating.) Make sure your hand is nice and warm. Baby may not appreciate a cold surprise.

Offer finger sucks. Nothing is more intimate than the first time your baby sucks on your little finger. Cut your fingernail short and scrub your pinky shiny clean. Place your finger against baby's cheek or lips, and baby may reflexively open her mouth and gently suck on your finger. Keep your face close to baby's in case she opens her eyes.

Give a quiet voice. Your baby can hear you and will become familiar with your voice. Quietly sing and talk to your baby. This will leave a lasting impression on her.

Be sure to ask the nurses if baby is ready for these activities. If you feel baby is ready but the nurses say no, discuss the reasons with the nurses and doctors. If any of these activities are too stimulating for your baby, don't worry. In another week or two she will probably welcome these sounds and touches from you.

Moderately Premature Babies

Babies between 30 and 34 weeks' gestational age will look more like full-term babies, only smaller. They move more because their nervous systems are more mature, although their movements continue to be uncoordinated and not purposeful. Baby's grasp will be stronger, and she can move her head from side to side. Your baby will begin to cry, a sound you've been waiting to hear. Baby will be awake more, with alert periods lasting several minutes. Baby will fix and focus on objects up to 8 to 10 inches away, such as your face. She will turn away from bright lights. Baby's suck will be more vigorous, and sucking on your finger or a pacifier can calm and comfort her.

Now that she is older and better able to handle stimulation, there are numerous ways you can become more physically involved with your baby. Keep in mind that your baby will still sleep most of the day. Ask your nurses if baby seems to have some regular, predictable times when she is awake and alert. Then be sure not to miss them!

Hold your baby. Once baby is off the ventilator (if she ever required one), you can finally hold her, a most rewarding parent-baby activity. Get comfortable in a rocking chair next to baby's crib, raise your feet up on a footstool, and ask the nurse to place baby into your welcoming arms. The skin-to-skin contact helps babies remain warm and stable. The nurse may want baby to stay attached to the monitors, but don't let this interfere with your enjoyment. As long as baby is happy and warm, there is really no limit to how long you can hold your baby this way. (See Practice Kangaroo Care, page 68, to read more about how babies benefit from this time.) If baby's heart rate, breathing pattern, or body temperature shows signs of instability, she will have to return to the isolette crib. As baby grows and the nurses become more confident that you can manage baby on your own, you can begin to pick up baby and hold her without assistance.

Talk to baby. When you talk or sing, baby may turn toward your voice. Even if you don't get this kind of response from baby, you can be sure your unique voice and speech patterns are imprinting themselves on baby's brain. She knows you're there and that you're important.

Star gaze. Your baby can focus clearly on your face. Get comfortable next to baby's crib on the side toward which his head is turned and just sit quietly and enjoy gazing at him. Speak softly and gently exaggerate your facial expressions. You may even notice that baby's gaze follows you as you slowly move to one side or the other.

Enjoy visual stimulation. Place a black-and-white-striped toy or picture in baby's crib. Baby's maturing vision responds well to dark-and-light contrasts.

We brought in a womb-sounds player, tape player, and a mobile. They let us have those in and on her bed.

Try infant massage. With increasing maturity, your baby will be able to tolerate, and even enjoy, more physical contact. Gently move your hand over every part of baby's body. (Do not rub or do a deep massage.) Daily physical touch has been shown to improve the growth and development of preemies.

We learned how to hand swaddle her to prevent added stress to her delicate little self.

Change diapers. As baby begins tube feedings, she will begin passing stools. While the nurses will certainly change your baby's diaper as part of their routine care, this is a place where you can jump in and do your part as much as you want.

Use your finger as a pacifier. You may find that your baby loves to suck. Your clean finger is still the most intimate pacifier short of the breast.

Enjoy feedings. Around 32 weeks of age, babies are able to suck more effectively, and you can finally begin to do what you have longed to do for weeks — feed your baby. (For instructions on breastfeeding and bottlefeeding your baby, see chapters 6, 7, and 8.)

Respect down time. You may see baby gets fussy and squirmy during playtime, a sign that he is feeling overstimulated and needs to be left alone for a while. Don't take this personally. Gently lay him back in his crib and try again later.

Mildly Premature Babies

Babies born between 35 and 37 weeks' gestation, especially those over 5 pounds,

---

DRESSING YOUR PREEMIE

When your preemie is on a warming bed or in an isolette, she will often be clad only in a diaper and cap. That's because it's easier to monitor and observe a mostly naked baby than one who is covered with clothing from head to toe. Babies also need to be bare when under a phototherapy lamp so that the jaundice-removing rays of light can reach baby's skin. As baby matures and emerges from the tubes and wires, you can start putting some clothes on baby. Begin with little socks. Unless your baby has an IV in her foot, these will not interfere with caregiving. Be sure any clothes you bring to the hospital for baby are soft (100 percent cotton) and loose-fitting. Wash new clothing in gentle detergent before putting it on your baby. Dressing baby up is a lot of fun for parents, since it reminds you that your baby is an individual. Forget proper fit. Little babies in big clothes brings a little humor into the NICU.

---

have mature lungs and nervous systems and often don't even need to go to the NICU. Most of these babies will move, cry, open their eyes, suck eagerly, and have longer alert periods. They are almost like full-term babies, and you can generally interact without restrictions. Some mildly premature babies weigh as little as 3½ to 4 pounds and may be more easily overstimulated. The guidelines in the preceding section offer suggestions for getting to know your baby slowly and gently.

HELPING BABY FEEL GOOD

Knowing what makes baby feel good is where parents really shine as part of the medical team. Get to know your baby's signs of distress and figure out what makes her feel more content. Keep notes: How does she like to be touched? What sounds does she like? In what position is she most comfortable? Your baby's preferences may change as she does. In general, preemies need small, frequent, and appropriate interactions rather than a whole lot of stimulation. The following are some parental preemie favorites:

Stroking baby's back. You may find that your preemie settles best when lying on her tummy or side, knees tucked under her in the fetal position. Maybe this reminds her of the comfort and security of the womb. Often preemies are positioned to sleep on their tummies, which helps them to breathe more easily. (This is safe to do in the hospital because baby is on a monitor.) They are encouraged to be on their backs when awake. When baby is relaxed, gently stroke her back or chest with the pads of your fingertips. Try to provide just the right amount of stimulation — not too much, not too little. You'll literally get a feel for which touches soothe your baby and which touches startle her.

Wrap your baby. Some babies enjoy the security of being wrapped tightly in a blanket. This is fine for a few hours from time to time. However, swaddling for long periods of time, such as all day and night, may lead to hip problems, even in term babies. Tight swaddling limits hip movement, which can prevent the hip joints from developing properly and lead to dislocation of the hip. Because of the increased incidence of hip dislocation in infants who are swaddled a lot, the custom of swaddling infants for prolonged periods of time has fallen out of favor.

Pacify baby. Sucking is soothing. Some ultrasound pictures show babies sucking their thumbs in the womb. Because sucking is calming, nurses often encourage a baby to suck during painful procedures, especially when blood is drawn from an artery to measure oxygen levels. Offer your baby a finger or a pacifier to suck during or after painful procedures. One day, baby will be ready to suck at Mom's breast for comfort during or after needle sticks.

Restore the peace. When the painful procedure is over, comfort your baby promptly. Do the best you can — by stroking, rocking, singing, or nursing — to help baby back into a more peaceful state. Think of yourself as baby's recovery doctor.

Hold your baby. Hold your baby as much as his medical condition allows. If baby is not yet ready to come out of the isolette, get your hands around as much of your baby as possible.

PROVIDE BREAST MILK FOR YOUR BABY

What would you say if your doctor told you this: "Besides caring for your baby's respiratory system, our two greatest challenges in the coming weeks are (1) to get his intestines to mature enough to handle milk feedings well, and (2) to protect him from infection. Any complications your baby has in these two areas could be life threatening and will prolong his stay in the NICU. There is medication we can give your baby that will help prevent these complications. Do you want us to give your baby that medicine?" Of course your answer would be a resounding "Yes!"

The "medicine" that will lessen your baby's risk of gastrointestinal problems and infection does not come from any large pharmaceutical company, and it costs very little to provide. The "medicine" is your breast milk. Giving your baby your milk is the single most important "therapeutic" thing you can do to help your preemie grow.

The most severe intestinal complication a preemie can have when feeding starts is necrotizing enterocolitis. NEC is described in detail in chapter 12, and how breast milk protects against NEC is detailed in chapter 6. But we would like to mention right now that research has shown that formula-fed preemies have a far greater chance of developing NEC than do breast milk–fed preemies.

Much of your baby's medical care in the weeks to come will focus on making sure baby's intestines are tolerating milk feedings, increasing the volume of feedings, watching baby gain weight, changing baby over to nipple feedings, and finally demonstrating that baby can thrive on nipple feedings alone. During these weeks in which baby's intestines are maturing, the medical staff will be hoping and praying that baby does not catch any infections. Despite all the hand washing and gown wearing everyone does, your baby will still be exposed to many germs during his time in the NICU, and his own natural immune system is just as immature as the rest of him. Nature has designed human milk to protect baby from infection until his own immune system can do the job by itself. Full-term babies need breast milk for this reason, and preemies need it even more. Research has made it clear that breast milk–fed preemies experience far fewer infections than do formula-fed preemies.

Your milk is so important to your baby that we have devoted two chapters (chapters 6 and 7) to this subject. We want you to have all the information you need to make breastfeeding work for you and your baby.

In the first days after a preemie is born, mothers must decide whether or not to begin pumping breast milk for baby. If your baby was born moderately to extremely premature and is on a ventilator machine, you may look at your sedated and fragile baby and realize that she is many weeks away from being able to suckle at your breasts. Further, the thought of pumping your breasts several times a day for many weeks, with no guarantee that baby will ever nurse at the breast, may be overwhelming. Why even start? When faced with the many challenges of spending time with your preemie, traveling to and from the hospital, taking care of other kids at home, and perhaps returning to work, you may worry that pumping breast milk will be too hard, or too stressful, or just one more thing that you have to juggle and feel inadequate about.

We ask you to look at this decision a little differently. Instead of deciding right now whether or not you want to face the many challenges of eventually breastfeeding your baby, make a decision to simply provide pumped breast milk for your baby right now — for the next week, or two, or three. You don't even need to make a decision about breastfeeding until your baby is actually ready to breastfeed. But your baby may be ready to start tube feedings now or within a matter of days. The doctors will need something to feed your baby. They will either use your breast milk, which is lovingly provided by your body and is a perfect nutritional match for your baby's premature needs, or they will use a manufactured substitute which is an adequate mix of nutrients but severely lacking in the myriad biological factors found in breast milk that promote your baby's intestinal and immunological development.

Your doctors may decide to start giving your baby feedings much sooner than you think. A technique called trophic feedings (also termed minimal enteral nutrition or GI priming) involves giving baby tiny amounts of milk through a feeding tube directly into the stomach starting in the first few days of life. This milk doesn't really provide much nutrition. Rather, it stimulates the stomach and intestines to mature faster and become better able to digest and absorb milk without any complications when full feedings are eventually started. Research has shown that babies who receive these early trophic

feedings fare better in the weeks to come and eventually tolerate full tube feedings faster than babies who don't get the "guts primed" for food.

Questions You May Have About Breast Milk

I am taking medications for postpartum complications, and my doctor says I can't breastfeed. What can I do?

Most postpartum complications, and the medications used to treat them, are only temporary. You can begin pumping and then discard your breast milk until you are off the medications. When you are well, you will have an abundant milk supply ready for your baby. Some mothers are actually given the wrong advice about a medication's incompatibility with breastfeeding. New research is done every year on a variety of drugs, and what was felt to be unsafe for baby through breast milk a few years ago may now be considered safe. Ask the lactation consultant to help you research this. (See Resources, page 235.)

While you "pump and dump" your breast milk, is formula the only option for your baby's feeds? No. Pasteurized donor breast milk has been used safely for many decades in NICUs and is a much healthier alternative to formula. See page 102 to read more about this option.

Many mothers find that the routine of pumping breast milk provides them with a comforting sense of involvement with their baby. They find that they are spending many hours in the NICU anyway, and using part of this time to pump becomes a welcome break from the routine of just sitting by baby's bedside.

If breast milk really can make such a difference, why doesn't everybody provide it for their premature babies?

Perhaps the biggest reason is lack of information. Everybody knows breast milk is better, but they may not know exactly how much better it is and why it is so special for preemies. Another reason is that during the initial days of having a premature baby, some parents feel they cannot make the time commitment and the emotional commitment to pumping and breastfeeding. They feel that they cannot add any more stress and worry to their lives. A third reason some parents may choose not to provide breast milk for their baby is that the medical staff does not offer enough support and information to help the mother get off to a good start with pumping. Or, the medical staff may hesitate to voice a strong opinion about something they regard as a strictly personal decision. However, because of the accumulation of studies showing improved outcomes in human milk–fed preemies, parents are now finding that doctors and nurses are more supportive of breastfeeding and that most NICUs have professional lactation consultants on staff.

BECOME FAMILIAR WITH YOUR BABY'S CARE

While we encourage parents of preemies to learn as much about their baby's medical care as they can, your most important job is to be your baby's mom or dad. Don't underestimate the importance of the simple things you do as baby's parent: providing physical touch and stimulation and being the one constant in the whirl-wind of caregivers surrounding baby's isolette.

Dr. Bill advises: The nurses and other medical staff are used to certain routines in the way they care for the preemies in the unit, but they know that every baby's needs change from day to day. The medical staff will welcome your observations and will use the information to personalize the care they give your baby. One of the first pieces of advice I give parents of preemies at their baby's bedside is this: "Become a keen observer and accurate reporter." During all aspects of your baby's care, especially during feedings, keep a watchful eye on what techniques work and which don't. Record them in a diary. The nurses must think about many babies at once, but you can focus on your baby alone. You will know what position makes breathing easiest for your baby and which feeding technique seems to be best tolerated. There will be days when she seems to grow better, sleep more soundly, and have fewer medical problems. You may be able to figure out what was different about her care those days. In watching parents at their preemie's bedside, I have noticed that they develop an intuitive sense of what kind of care will work best for their baby.

Be your baby's advocate. Your many hours of being with your baby give you an intuitive sense of baby's progress, whether for better or worse. Mother's intuition depends heavily on an accumulation of information in your brain that allows you to "just know" what's going on with your baby.

Now, we don't want you to sound the alarm over every tiny bump on baby's

---

AS YOUR BABY GROWS, KEEP A JOURNAL

Don't let your wisdom and your observations about your baby go unrecorded. While at your baby's bedside, you'll have plenty of time to keep a journal. Write down your fears, hopes, and dreams, and record day-to-day happenings. Write down what seems to agitate your baby and what works best to keep your baby comfortable. Describe any special care he received on his best days, and you will eventually develop your own wisdom that you can share with the nurses about "what works." Leave room in the journal for pictures. Write down valuable tips from the nurses. When you get your baby home, you will forget a lot of what you learned in the NICU and you will find this written record very helpful. Don't let what you're learning go to waste.

If you prefer using a laptop to writing with paper and pencil, you can keep an electronic journal, complete with digital pictures. You can share parts of your journal online with friends and family.

I wish I had taken more pictures of my daughter when she was first born, even in those very early days when she was red and skinny. They fill out so fast, and it's hard to remember how tiny she really was.

---

skin, every hiccup, every sneeze, or every half teaspoon of spit-up. But we do want you to be a parent who does not hesitate to stand up for your baby when your intuition tells you something is not quite right.

By spending time holding and touching your baby and educating yourself about your baby's care, you may become the best monitor that baby has.

Practice the art of advice giving. There are three different ways parents typically voice their worries. There is timid Tim, who quietly says, "I know I don't know much, and my baby's probably fine, but I think there might be something wrong." Demanding Dana puts it this way: "I am my baby's mother, and I know I'm right! I insist that you go get the doctor this second!" Patient Pauline has been practicing her powers of suggestion, gets her nurse's attention, places a gentle hand on the nurse's arm, and says in a confident tone, "I appreciate the close attention you pay to my baby. I need your help in deciding something with me. Can you come take a look at baby's skin and tell me if this new rash, which I didn't notice yesterday, is of any concern?" Pauline displays several important communication skills that will ensure her concerns are heard:

- *Radiate confidence.* When someone senses that you feel sure about your concern, he or she may pay closer attention.
- *Start with a compliment.* This is a good way to approach people in any walk of life. When you let people know that you trust them, they will be more receptive. It doesn't have to be a big compliment, but it should be genuine.
- *Try touch.* If you feel it's appropriate, a gentle hand on the arm or shoulder creates more of a connection between you and your listener.
- *Ask for help.* You will get much farther with the phrase "I need your help" than

you will with "I demand you listen to me." Doctors and nurses are very accustomed to helping when asked. They want to help people. That's why they went into this profession.

- *Mention that you have been spending time with baby, observing him closely.* Put your question in the context of your many observations about your baby: "This rash wasn't here yesterday" or "He's so much more awake today."

- *Be careful about your timing.* Asking your nurse to check on a minor problem with your baby while she is engaged in a major procedure with another baby not only won't work but it's also inconsiderate. In addition, when you repeatedly demand immediate attention for small issues, you may not be taken seriously if something really important comes up.

We don't want you to be afraid of the medical staff or feel that you must have the diplomatic skills of an ambassador to the UN to communicate with doctors and nurses. Most of these communication tips are only common courtesies. This is the way you talk to friends, coworkers, or business associates. But when your own tiny baby is the focus of your communication, your emotions can make it harder to speak your mind in a tactful way. NICU staff members understand this, but they will find it easier to communicate with you if you practice good communication skills with them.

PRACTICE KANGAROO CARE

Kangaroo care — holding your preemie skin-to-skin — is one of the best ways you can get involved in helping your preemie thrive. Kangaroo care gets its name from the way a mother kangaroo cares for her tiny baby joey. Just as the kangaroo mother's pouch gives her baby a safe, protected environment close to her body but outside the womb, kangaroo care in the NICU puts preemies in the most natural place possible — between Mother's breasts. Practicing K care is where parents can really shine. Here's why it's good for baby — and for Mom and Dad.

As with so many other surprising medical advances, necessity was the mother of invention that led to kangaroo care. The medical benefits of skin-to-skin holding for preemies were discovered quite by chance in the early 1980s by two neonatologists in Bogotá, Colombia. Because their hospitals couldn't afford enough modern high-tech isolettes for preemies, they used what they had to hold and warm tiny babies — the babies' mothers, a low-tech but high-touch solution. The premature baby was placed skin-to-skin on Mother's chest, between her breasts. A cloth wrapped around Mother's body

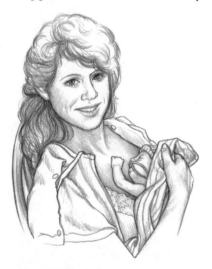

held baby there (originally this custom was dubbed "packing"). The mothers were instructed to hold their infants twenty-four hours a day, sleep with them, and let the baby suckle from the breast. Babies were even given oxygen while nestled on mother's chest. Dramatic improvements occurred in the "kangarooed" preemies. Not only did more preemie babies survive, but they thrived better: infants gained weight faster and left the hospital sooner. It took an experiment of necessity in poor hospitals in South America to demonstrate how important parental care is to premature infants. Gradually, kangaroo care has become more popular, and researchers have learned that it provides substantial benefits for babies, even in the high-tech hospitals of Europe and North America.

Babies grow better. Remember, your goal is not just for your baby to grow heavier and taller, but also to mature physically, emotionally, and intellectually. One reason kangarooed babies gain weight faster is that they are able to conserve energy when held against mother's chest. Crying, fussing, exhibiting stress, and trying to stay warm use up calories that babies need to grow. Because K-care babies cry less, fuss less, are less stressed, and have more stable body temperatures, they waste fewer calories and are able to use these extra calories to grow.

Another reason K-care babies grow better is that they feed better. Studies show that when babies spend many hours nestled next to the breast and are allowed to suck at their own pace (called self-regulatory feeding), mothers enjoy a more efficient milk-ejection reflex and deliver more milk. Put smart babies next to their milk supply and naturally they're going to nurse more.

K-care babies also thrive better because

SCIENCE SAYS "KANGAROOED" BABIES THRIVE BETTER

Many scientists have shown the following benefits of kangaroo care to parents and preemies.

Preemies	Parents (especially mothers)
• gain weight faster • leave the hospital sooner • cry less • have more stable temperatures • are more alert • sleep better • breathe better • have more stable heart rates	• are less depressed • are more comfortable in the NICU • are more confident in caregiving ability • have a more positive attitude toward baby • perceive baby as less abnormal • interact more with baby • feel more important • bond better

they are calmer. Research shows that K-care babies have lower levels of stress hormones than babies who are separated frequently from their mothers.

K-care babies also sleep better. Growth hormone is secreted during sleep, so it stands to reason that the more restful the sleep, the better the growth. The reasons that kangaroo care promotes growth can be summed up in one word: "organizing." The close contact with the mother helps the baby's body systems mature and become more organized. When these systems work more efficiently, baby grows more quickly. (For more on organizing a preemie's physiology, see page 164.)

Babies breathe better. Research has shown that K-care babies have higher blood oxygen levels and require supplemental oxygen less often than when in an incubator. They also have fewer apnea episodes. Wouldn't it be nice to get your baby off that nasal oxygen tube?

It promotes bonding. Kangaroo care enables you to get a feel for your baby's body and behavior and, above all, learn to read her cues. As you are rocking, holding, and nursing your baby, imagine you are empowering her to grow and thrive as you enfold her with your love. This skin-to-skin contact with your baby actually makes you feel closer to her. You don't just love her with your mind, you love her with your body. Mothers' bodies respond to K-care by producing more of the breastfeeding hormones prolactin and oxytocin. These hormones produce feelings of relaxation and love, and these good feelings reinforce your instinct to care for your baby. Because holding your

baby feels nice, you want to hold her more and more, and the more you hold her, the more confident you feel about your ability to care for her.

It reduces pain response. New research has shown that preemies feel less pain during procedures such as heel sticks when held in the K-care position before and during the procedure. Ask the nurse to allow you to assist in this manner when appropriate.

K-care babies leave the hospital sooner. Because kangaroo-care babies grow faster, breathe better, and feed better, they are discharged from the NICU, and the hospital, sooner. In some studies, kangarooed preemies were found to enjoy a 50 percent shorter hospital stay. Insurance companies take note: Pay the "kangaroo" mom!

It protects babies from infection. One worry that medical personnel have about taking a preemie out of the "sterile" isolette is that exposing baby to more germs through skin-to-skin contact may give him an infection. However, research has shown K care does not increase infection rates in babies. As parents spend more and more time at baby's bedside, they are exposed to the natural bacteria that dwell around baby in the NICU. Research has shown that Mom will start producing antibodies to these germs, and baby will then get these antibodies through the breast milk. What better way to protect baby! (Infections caused by germs that live in the NICU are called nosocomial infections. These are a constant threat to preemies, and anything that can be done to decrease this risk will benefit baby.)

PARENTS AS PACEMAKERS

While you've probably never thought of yourself as a breathing machine or a heart rate monitor, that's essentially what you are when you hold your baby close to you. Studies have shown that when babies nestle against a parent's chest, especially with their ear over the heartbeat, the contact with the parent's body seems to stabilize the baby's breathing and heart rate.

Preemies' ability to regulate their own breathing is very immature. They frequently have stop-breathing episodes, a problem called apnea, for fifteen or twenty seconds at a time. When they don't breathe, their blood oxygen gets low and their heart rate goes down. Frequent apnea episodes are hard on baby and interfere with growth.

When baby is snuggled comfortably against your chest with her ear over your heart, the rhythm of your breathing, your heartbeat, your voice, your movement, and even the warm air you exhale from your nose onto baby's scalp all provide natural stimuli that "remind" the "forgetful" preemie to breathe. Little bodies that have more stable heart and breathing rates thrive better.

Contact with a parent also helps baby maintain a stable body temperature. Preemies' immature nervous systems have trouble regulating their temperature, and preemies get cold easily because they don't have the layer of fat that is deposited under the skin in the late weeks of pregnancy.

When you put baby skin-to-skin with a warm mommy or daddy, his body temperature usually remains stable. A fascinating study demonstrated a "thermal synchrony" between mother and baby during kangaroo care. When a K-care baby's temperature went down, the mother's temperature went up, especially the skin temperature of her breasts, and she warmed up her baby. This phenomenon is just one more example of how a mother's physiology provides for the extra needs of her preemie. Her special milk contains the added nutrients her baby needs and protects baby from infection. Her body can help him cope with the problems of having an immature nervous system.

Dr. Bob advises: While you are holding your baby near your breast, take a moment to note baby's oxygen levels and other readings on the various monitors. Notice if they get better when baby is held against your body. (They usually do!) Occasionally when a preemie is moved from the crib to Mom's arms, baby's vital signs and oxygen levels will fluctuate for the worse. This is probably temporary. Don't panic and rush baby back into the isolette and feel like your bonding experiment has failed. Be patient. Let baby get settled with you. If the vital signs don't improve, then put baby back and try again later.

How to do it. While there are different styles for different kangaroo pairs, here

SCIENCE SAYS: KANGAROO-CARE BABIES AND PARENTS BECOME MORE CONNECTED

A 2002 study comparing seventy-three K-care preemies with seventy-three preemies receiving standard care showed that at six months, K-care infants and their parents were more connected. The K-care infants scanned the mother's face more, interacted with her more, and were generally more alert during interactions. They were also more attentive and showed better exploratory skills. The K-care mothers felt more positive toward their infants and looked at and interacted with them more. K-care mothers were less depressed and regarded their infants as more "normal." Both mothers and fathers in the K-care group were more responsive to their infant's needs and more adept at reading their infant's cues.

Researchers theorize that the greater responsiveness to their babies in K-care mothers was due, at least in part, to biology. The contact with their babies increased the women's levels of hormones oxytocin and prolactin. These hormones are involved in the production and delivery of milk to the baby, and they also seem to be the biological basis of mother's intuition. The hormonal boost that mothers received during kangaroo care may have made them more sensitive, warm, and adaptive. The researchers also theorized that K-care babies were more alert and attentive with their mothers, and this in turn brought out more maternal behavior in the mother.

The K-care infants scored higher on developmental tests, and interestingly, the differences between groups in motor development were greatest in the preemies with the highest level of risk. Researchers suggest that the sickest and youngest preemies are most in need of kangaroo care and will benefit the most from it.

Quite a system, isn't it? Babies help mothers to be better mothers, and mothers help babies to be better babies.

are some general tips that work for most preemies and their parents:

- While each NICU has its own policy about kangaroo care, you can usually begin as soon as baby is off the ventilator. Many NICUs try to have parents begin kangaroo care as early as four hours after baby's birth.
- Get a comfortable chair, preferably a reclining chair with a footrest. Some nurseries have special chairs just for kangaroo care. Rocking chairs also work well.

- Wear comfortable clothing and a blouse that opens easily in the front. Remove your bra to allow for maximum skin-to-skin contact. A nurse will help you and your baby get comfortable as you are learning K care.
- Dress baby only in a diaper and a cap. Place baby between your breasts with his head turned to the side, ear over your heart, and his mouth at nipple level. Baby's chest and abdomen are skin-to-skin with yours. Drape a blanket or wrap your blouse or sweater over baby's back.

- Relax and enjoy! Baby needs to sense how relaxed you are. Rock slowly and rhythmically. Sing a lullaby. Let baby suck as she desires. The first few attempts at K care are practice time as you get to know what is most comfortable for you and your baby. Try not to overstimulate baby, especially in the beginning, by rocking, singing, and nursing all at the same time. Let baby concentrate on one thing at a time. When he's older, he will enjoy more input from you.
- As you and your baby are getting used to K care, the nurse may check baby's temperature frequently. Chances are, your baby will not have trouble maintaining a stable body temperature when held against your skin. Mother is a much better infant warmer than the mechanical incubator is. As a testimony to how nature intends mothers and babies to enjoy frequent skin-to-skin contact, if baby's body temperature drops, Mom's skin temperature will rise, to warm him up again. (Some of the warmest organs of your body — your liver and your breasts — are close to baby's skin.)
- Dads, too! Mothers are usually the first to try kangaroo care. Once Dad sees how well it is working, he'll be more confident and comfortable about joining the fun. As much as possible, share the K care. Dads can't breastfeed, but they can soothe and comfort with touch and closeness. In fact, one unique advantage for dad is that the lower-pitched male voice creates more soothing vibrations as he snuggles baby's head against the front of his neck and drapes his chin over the top of baby's head (a comforting technique we dubbed the neck nestle).

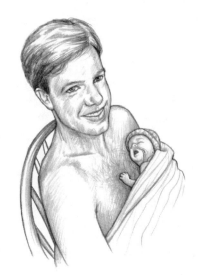

- Enlist the nurses as coaches. Try to find out which nurses are the most experienced and supportive of kangaroo care and ask for their help.
- Try K care for at least three hours a day while in the hospital and for many more hours the first few months at home.
- Once baby is detached from tubes and wires and in the "grower" nursery, you can practice kangaroo care while walking around and wearing your baby in a sling. This is more like the real kangaroo pouch!

What helps all babies, especially preemies, thrive? Better sleep, stable temperature and breathing, and better food. Kangaroo care gives baby all three. Kangaroo care works because it makes good physiological sense. Preemies get short-changed on time in the womb, but K care provides an "outside womb." (For more on the physiological benefits of baby-wearing, see page 150.)

A HAPPY BED!

One worry many parents have is whether or not their baby is happy when they are not around to hold and comfort him. They imagine their baby being left to fuss and cry sometimes because the nurse is busy providing medical care to several other babies. As your baby gets older and more aware, his needs for comforting throughout the day and night may increase. The nurses truly do their best to care for all the babies, but they might not be able to tend to your baby every second that your baby cries. Many NICUs have nurse's aides and hospital volunteers who come in to hold fussy babies and help with feeding and other routine tasks.

Some NICUs and pediatric hospitals keep babies happy when unattended by using a baby hammock device invented in Australia that has recently been introduced to U.S. hospitals and homes. Called the Amby Baby Motion Bed, this bassinet hangs suspended from a steel frame by a sturdy spring and crossbar. Every little movement your baby makes creates a gentle bouncing and rocking motion that soothes her just as if she were being rocked in a caregiver's arms. The Amby Bed has several features that make it ideal for preemies:

It provides a continuum of the womb environment. The Amby Bed gently moves baby both up and down and from side to side, creating the same simultaneous bouncing and swinging motion that baby experienced while inside the womb and when carried in your arms. This gives baby a greater sense of well-being and contentment when left unattended.

It lessens acid reflux. By keeping baby slightly upright, this hammock minimizes painful acid heartburn and reduces the amount of milk your baby spits up (see Gastroesophageal Reflux Disease, page 195).

It may reduce apnea and bradycardia. One of the most common causes of apnea and bradycardia (long pauses in breathing and slowed heart rate, respectively) is acid reflux, which irritates baby's breathing passage and can trigger apnea spells.

It helps baby grow. Baby fusses less, so he uses more of his energy for growth. Baby also spits up less milk, so he has more to grow on.

It provides continued kangaroo care when you are not there. Research has demonstrated the benefits of kangaroo care (see page 68). Nothing helps baby thrive better than being held skin-to-skin in your arms. But when you can't be there, this hammock gives your baby a womblike environment to thrive in.

(See page 161 for illustration and information on home use. You can read more about the Amby Baby Motion Bed at www.AmbyBaby.com.)

DECORATE YOUR PREEMIE'S HOSPITAL "NURSERY"

If your baby is going to be in the special care nursery for several weeks or even months, you might as well try to make it feel like home.

Dim the lights. Remember the womb is a very dark environment, and flashing lights on monitors and harsh fluorescent lights overhead are new, stressful experiences for a preemie. Many newborn specialists feel that the bright fluorescent lights in hospitals cause sensory overload in preemies. For this reason, many nurseries provide a cover for baby's isolette, which darkens baby's surroundings and blocks out upsetting stimulation. If your nursery does not provide such a cover, make your own from fabric. Choose colors that you enjoy looking at, because you're going to be looking at it a lot. Experts differ over whether it's better for premature babies to rest in darkness most of the day and night or only at night. The advantage of night darkness only is that baby gets introduced to the day/night cycle of his new world.

We encouraged dimming the lights at night when the staff was used to leaving them on.

Mute the noise. Not only are premature babies' eyes sensitive to bright lights, but their ears are bothered by loud noises. You will notice that your baby startles in reaction to loud noises. Startling is a reflex in which baby's arms and legs are suddenly flung out to the sides, away from his body. Sometimes you'll notice that the oxygen saturation level goes down a bit following a startle, as it does in response to other stressful events, such as when babies are crying. The womb is certainly not a sound-free environment, but the sounds your baby heard in the womb — your heartbeat, the sound of blood whooshing through the arteries, and bowel sounds — were muted by the tissues of the womb and abdomen. Your baby's isolette is far from a noise-free environment, and the NICU is full of irritating noises that may bother your growing baby. Try these tips to make baby's NICU surroundings sound more like the womb:

- The thick isolette cover that you use to dim the light in the isolette can also mute the noise.
- Shut isolette doors, portholes, and nearby cabinet doors *quietly*.
- Don't place bottles or toys on the isolette, since they rattle and increase the noise inside.
- Avoid tapping or banging on the isolette yourself and caution baby's siblings not to do so.

A THERAPEUTIC VOICE

Make tape recordings of your voice talking and singing lullabies to your baby. You will naturally speak and sing in a loving way that no one else can. Studies have shown that babies, especially preemies, prefer the familiar voices of their parents over the voices of strangers. Record a medley of your favorite lullabies and set up the tape recorder to play them continuously for baby.

- Speak softly to your baby in a gentle, high, light voice. Remind visitors to speak softly when at baby's bedside.
- Play soothing music. Obviously, you should avoid playing loud music or blaring the radio in the NICU. Continuous, gentle, quiet music can calm baby and also be comforting to you during the many hours at your baby's bedside. Bring tapes or CDs and something to play them on, as well as headphones. Remember, this will be your "home" for a while, too. Make it as pleasant as you can.
- A music box playing a soothing lullaby is a welcome addition to your baby's "nursery" and welcome to your baby's ears — and yours.

Hang mementos. Since this is also going to be your home away from home for weeks or months, decorate it with things that make you feel good. Display photos of your other children or of family and friends, or hang a sequence of photos tracing your preemie's growth along the wall next to the incubator. If a relative or a friend has made something special for baby, or if you have been working on a project in the NICU, display this, too.

Leave a bit of yourself behind. To help your baby connect with mother's natural body scent, leave one of your nursing bras, or a pad that has been in your bra, in the corner of the isolette. Studies show that newborn babies are drawn to their mother's scent more than to a stranger's scent.

Bring toys for tiny tots. It's okay for friends, relatives, and siblings to bring a few special toys for baby. You certainly don't want to stuff the isolette with toys, and really, your baby couldn't care less

about them. (He just wants to eat, sleep, grow, and get out of there!) But toys and teddy bears make baby's surroundings look more like a real nursery. A cute teddy bear propped next to the isolette adds a bit of comfort and makes it easier for parents and medical staff to cope with an otherwise stressful and technologically sterile environment.

Here's an idea for a toy that baby *can* play with, once she is in the "grower" nursery and her eyes are open most of the time. A mirror placed about 12 inches from her eyes will give her something interesting to look at (herself!) that is not too stimulating. (Preemies see objects most clearly at a distance of 12 inches.)

Minimize disturbances. Preemies who remain calm breathe better and grow faster. Do the best you can to minimize intrusions. You can request that a test or procedure be delayed for an hour or two if possible so that baby can sleep longer. The nurses will try to do most necessary procedures at one time, when baby is awake. This is called cluster care, and it ensures that babies are allowed long periods of undisturbed sleep, which is important to their growth. But it is not always possible to avoid waking baby. It's also important that you limit your playful interactions with baby to times when he is in the state of quiet alertness, the behavioral state in which babies are most interactive. Don't stimulate a baby who needs to sleep.

TAKE GOOD CARE OF YOURSELF

In the first days of your baby's life in the NICU, it is natural to want to be by her side every minute. After all, these may be the most challenging weeks of her life, and you want to be with her through it all. By the time you have read this far in this book, you have probably already realized that even the most dedicated parent can't stay at baby's bedside twenty-four hours a day. Even twelve-hour shift work with a spouse will quickly leave you both physically and emotionally exhausted. In this state, you can't help your baby. Your baby needs you healthy, happy, and well rested. A baby can sense how her parents are feeling. A positive, involved, energetic parent will provide a higher level of care and emotional support to baby than will a worn-out, depressed, half-asleep parent, however dedicated and well intentioned. You may be able to keep up an all-day and all-night vigil in the NICU for a couple days during critical periods, but we encourage you to listen to the medical staff when they urge you to go home and rest. Here are some ways that you can spend the most quality time with your baby while taking good care of yourself:

Eat well. Good nutrition will give you more energy. It will keep your immune system healthier so that you are less likely to get sick. (If you get sick, you won't be allowed to get close to baby.) Good nutrition also helps breastfeeding mothers' milk supply. Stay away from fast-food meals. The convenience is tempting, but high-fat, low-nutrient burgers, fries, and chicken will leave you feeling sluggish. Bring healthy snacks, such as nuts and dried fruit, to the NICU. Ask friends to bring some easily warmed-up meals to your house (casseroles are quick and easy) so you can enjoy fast, but home-cooked, meals.

Sleep well. You will quickly learn how valuable sleep is. Too little sleep not only

---

TAKING CARE OF YOURSELF WHILE TAKING CARE OF BABY

When your baby is hospitalized, all your worry and concern is for her. You stay with her, you hold her, you nurse her, you comfort her, and you worry. You may forget to eat or drink, or you may fail to sleep well. Your baby needs a healthy mother now more than ever. Here are some suggestions:

- Carry a water bottle and healthy snacks with you at all times.
- Wear comfortable lightweight clothes that make it easy to nurse or pump.
- Sleep when your baby sleeps. To minimize unnecessary interruptions, hang a PLEASE DO NOT DISTURB BABY OR MOTHER sign on baby's crib when you are napping.
- Arrange to have an electric breast pump at your baby's bedside.
- Talk to the nurses about getting food trays for yourself at mealtimes. The hospital staff can tell you where to get juice and snacks between meals. Since you are baby's food source, the hospital should feed your baby by feeding you.

Do your best to recover physically. Your baby will need you to be strong at home, when the nurses will not be caring for him 24/7.

---

robs you and baby of needed energy, but it can also lower your resistance to germs and make you susceptible to colds or flu. If you live far away from the hospital, find

SIBLING CARE AND INVOLVEMENT

Finding time for your baby in the NICU is even more challenging when you have other children at home. How do you divide your time appropriately? Here are some tips:

Ask for help. That's what family and close friends are for. Arrange for them to help with your little ones at home. If your NICU allows it, you can have close family members take shifts with the baby while you stay connected with your kids at home. Grandma and Grandpa especially may benefit from this bonding time with their preemie grandchild.

Young children age three and under may not understand that their new little brother or sister is sick and in the hospital. The new baby may not be real to them until he or she finally comes home. Yet, even young children sense your anxiety and know that something troubling has occurred in the family. They need to know why you are tired and have to be away from home a lot. Answer any questions you can. Let your child's questions be your guide to how much he or she needs to know. Complicated answers may make your child even more anxious.

Show and tell. Children four and older will have a better understanding that their little brother or sister was born but is not coming home yet. Answer questions and offer explanations on a level appropriate for your child. Show siblings pictures of "their" baby. You need not tell them the exact seriousness of baby's condition. Simple statements such as, "Baby has to stay in the hospi-

out if you can sleep at a friend's house who lives closer. Another option is to stay in a nearby inexpensive hotel a couple nights each week to avoid a long drive every day. The hospital social worker may be able to arrange accommodations for you near the hospital.

Feel good. A daily bath or shower and clean clothes rejuvenate tired bodies and spirits. Take the time to allow yourself these luxuries. You will feel better and be a better parent for your baby.

Get outside. When you take a break at the hospital, try to go outside. Ask the nurses for tips on nice places to go — a courtyard, a garden, a sidewalk café, a nearby park. Use this place for a little retreat during lunch or break time. Getting some fresh air and sunshine every day will help you cope better with the hospital atmosphere.

Get moving. Daily exercise helps boost your immune system and your "coping" systems. Explore where you can take a daily twenty- to thirty-minute brisk walk while baby is sleeping.

Talk to people. Make friends with the nurses, other parents, and social workers in the NICU. Some friendly conversation will lift your spirits and also help those tal for a while, and Mommy and Daddy get to be there a lot to feed and help baby grow" will help kids realize why you have to be gone so much.

Promote sibling bonding. Encourage your children to draw pictures and pick out gifts (e.g., a music box) for their little baby. Hang this art on or near baby's isolette. Take a picture of baby with big brother's art in the background. Let siblings pick out clothes and help you shop for baby's homecoming.

Encourage hospital visits. Some NICUs don't allow children to visit because of the belief that children are more likely to bring germs into the unit. However, there is no research to support this belief. Allowing sibling visitation probably does not increase the rate of infection in the NICU, provided chil-dren follow the same hygienic proce-dures adult visitors do. If you think it is appropriate, bring your children to the hospital to any available viewing area from which they might at least be able to see their baby sibling. You might also see if the baby can be brought to a visit-ing area for some family time. Of course, if children are sick, they should not enter the NICU.

Before taking your child to visit the baby, consider whether the high-tech atmosphere may be too frightening. You want her to come home from this visit reassured, not scared and worried. Pre-pare your child for the sights and sounds of the NICU, with photos or age-appropriate descriptions. The nurses in the NICU may be able to give you books or pamphlets to help explain your baby's care to your other children.

around you. Give yourself a break and talk about things other than your baby.

Support your spouse. The stress of hav-ing a premature baby can take its toll on a marriage. Take time daily to talk, hug, cry, and laugh together. Keep a close eye on your significant other. If you see signs of depression or burnout, talk about it with your spouse and help him or her figure out what to do to feel less stressed.

My husband and I devised our own "shift." Dad would visit for an hour on his way to work and again on his way home in the evening. I would arrive in the morn-ing and stay through the afternoon. We both got to know the day and evening nurses.

Enjoy family time. You and your partner are probably already taking shifts with baby. Instead of just taking turns at the hospital one at a time, enjoy some family time together with baby, as you would do if you were all at home. Such precious time will keep you better connected. Ad-ditionally, be sure to spend some time together at home with each other and with your other children. Take a break from the hospital and go out for dinner or a movie.

II

FEEDING YOUR PREEMIE

During the first year, preemies need more food, even though their intestines are not yet mature enough to digest the food as well as a term baby can. Naturally, this presents a challenge to parents. The goal in feeding your preemie is to give baby more for less: more milk, but less work while feeding. In this section, you will learn why breast milk is best for premature infants. You will learn about breastfeeding and bottlefeeding techniques and how to meet your preemie's extra nutritional needs. You will also learn how to feed infants who have a variety of common medical problems. Since you will spend more time feeding your baby than in any other single interaction during the early months, we want you and your baby to enjoy it.

Mother's Milk — The Perfect Food for Preemies!

DURING THE FIRST WEEKS of your preemie's life, the doctors and nurses will be doing everything they can to help your baby grow and develop. Yet there is one important thing that only you can do: give your baby your milk. Breast milk is more than nourishment for preemies: we call it M&Ms — mom's milk as medicine.

When a baby is born preterm, she doesn't get all the special nutrients that most babies receive through the placenta in the late months of pregnancy. Human milk provides these nutrients — and much more.

WHY MOTHER'S MILK IS SO SPECIAL FOR PREEMIES

Human milk is the "gold standard" of infant nutrition for full-term babies. Commercial infant formulas simply cannot duplicate the milk made by nature. When you deliver a premature baby, nature actually improves on itself, and mothers' breasts make a milk that contains even more of the special nutrients preemies need and would be getting if they were still in the womb.

Mothers of preemies make supermilk! Here are some of the special advantages of giving your preemie your milk:

SUPERMILK!

By a fortunate quirk of nature, mothers of preemies make milk that contains greater amounts of most of the nutrients that preemies need and in greater amounts than when they deliver full-term babies. It's as if your body makes "personal milk" for your baby! Research shows that preterm milk is higher in the following:

- calories
- fats
- proteins
- white blood cells
- immunoglobulins
- zinc
- calcium
- phosphorus

MOM'S MILK — THE PERFECT MATCH FOR HER PREEMIE	
Preemie Problems	**Mom's Milk as Medicine**
slow growth	has extra protein, fat, and calories
susceptibility to infection	has high doses of immune boosters and infection fighters
agitation, restlessness	relaxes baby
constipation	exerts laxative effect
immature digestion	is easiest to digest
catch-up brain growth	has special nutrients to help brain growth
intestinal inflammation (NEC)	protects against NEC
visual problems	improves visual acuity
breathing problems	is easier to breathe while breastfeeding than while bottlefeeding
weaker bones	builds stronger bones
anemia (low iron in the blood)	builds better blood
unstable body temperature	feeding at breast stabilizes body temperature
dry, flaky, sensitive skin	gives smoother, healthier skin
need for happy, relaxed mother	relaxes mother, boosts her confidence

Feeling important? You are!

Builds brighter brains. A baby's brain grows faster in the last trimester of pregnancy than at any other time of life. In fact, the brain of a 28-week preemie will double its weight in the next 8 weeks. Critical brain growth continues after birth, and human milk delivers the special nutrients needed to build better brains. A flurry of breast milk research over the past decade has shown that breastfed babies tend to grow up smarter, and this advantage of breastfeeding shows especially in preemies. A study in England compared preemies who were fed expressed human milk with those fed standard infant formulas. A follow-up of these babies at 18 months and again at eight years showed that the human milk–fed babies scored higher on developmental scales, and as a group they showed an IQ that was an average of 8.3 points higher. The more breast milk babies received, the better their scores. The infants in this study received human milk by tube feedings during the first 4 weeks of life. This and other features of the study design suggest that the human milk–fed babies were smarter because of specific nutrients in breast milk rather than differences in socioeconomic status or parenting practices between mothers who chose to pump milk for their babies and those who didn't. Researchers concluded there must be something special in mother's milk that enhances brain growth. Many other studies in recent years have also found that children who were breastfed show higher-than-average scores on developmental tests than children who were formula-fed.

The most likely candidates for the brain-building role of mother's milk are the "smart proteins" and "smart fats." Brain-boosting proteins include the amino acid taurine, which is present in much larger amounts in human milk than in formula. It is essential for optimal brain growth.

The "smart fats" are known as LC-PUFAs (pronounced "elsie-poofahs," which stands for long-chain polyunsaturated fatty acids). These include the fats called DHA (docosa-hexaenoic acid) and ARA (arachidonic acid), substances baby's body needs to make myelin, the fatty sheath that insulates nerves so that they can transmit messages faster and more efficiently. Getting enough LC-PUFAs is important for preemies for two reasons. First, it helps their immature brain grow fast, just like it would have in the womb. Second, preemies may not yet be able to manufacture sufficient LC-PUFAs on their own from other dietary fats. They need ready-made DHA and other smart fats from mother's milk. Colostrum, the yellow-gold milk made by mothers' breasts in the first days after baby's birth, is especially rich in smart fats, and levels of these fats remain high throughout the first month — just the time when your preemie needs them most.

Promotes better vision. Not only does breast milk build brighter brains, but it also builds better eyes. Studies comparing breastfed and formula-fed infants show that visual development is better in breast-fed babies, and these benefits are even more noticeable in premature infants. This makes sense, since the retina is made of nerve tissue, just like the brain. The same smart fats in breast milk that nourish the brain also help the retina develop. Other nutrients that are found in greater amounts in breast milk, such as beta carotene, taurine, and vitamin E, may also contribute to visual health. Give your preemie your milk to help your baby grow up to have a healthier "outlook" on life.

In addition, preemies who experience breathing difficulties may be exposed to prolonged high concentrations of oxygen. While the oxygen helps them breathe more easily, it can damage the immature retina. Breast milk helps protect against

---

SCIENCE SAYS: BREASTFED PREEMIES BECOME SMARTER KIDS

A review of twenty research studies concluded breastfed babies scored higher on intellectual testing as children and adolescents compared with formula-fed kids. The lower the birth weight, the greater the difference.

this damage. (See Retinopathy of Prematurity, page 200).

Helps preemies grow. Breast milk also helps build healthier bodies. Mothers of preemies produce milk that is higher in many nutrients that help their babies grow, especially fats, proteins, and calories. Studies show that breastfed preemies enjoy stronger bones, greater weight gain, and faster catch-up growth. Breast milk is rich in various growth factors, such as epidermal growth factor, insulinlike growth factor, and nerve growth factor. All of these help vital tissues and organs of the body develop, especially the brain, lungs, intestines, neural pathways, and skin. Also, the skin-to-skin contact, cuddling, and closeness that are naturally a part of breastfeeding help preemies stay calm and organized, and less stress means more energy devoted to growth and development.

Dr. Jim suggests: Try the taste test. Sample a bit of your pumped milk, then ask one of the nurses to give you a teaspoonful of the infant formula they usually use for preemies. If you were your baby, which would you want to drink?

SCIENCE SAYS: BREASTFED BABIES SEE BETTER

Research showed 50 percent less (and less severe) retinopathy of prematurity in breast milk–fed preemies compared with formula-fed preemies. There were some benefits in even partially breast milk–fed preemies.

SCIENCE SAYS: BREASTFED BABIES GO HOME SOONER

Breast milk–fed preemies leave the hospital earlier than those who are formula-fed. One study showed that breast milk–fed preemies stayed in the NICU an average of thirty-three days, whereas formula-fed preemies stayed an average of forty-one days. Another study showed that breast milk–fed preemies went home an average of fifteen days sooner than formula-fed preemies did.

Protects against infection. One of the most important reasons you should breastfeed your preemie is to reap the benefits of breast milk's ability to protect your baby from infection.

Shortly after birth, all babies acquire two types of germs, some potentially harmful and some healthful, that enter the intestines and take up residence there. A competition ensues between the concentrations of healthful and harmful bacteria. The healthful bacteria help to keep the harmful ones in check. Various substances in breast milk encourage the growth of healthful resident bacteria, especially lactobacilli.

Meanwhile, colostrum, the golden supermilk that you produce during the first week after baby is born, helps baby fight off harmful germs. As a perk, colostrum from mothers of preemies contains even higher concentrations of infection fighters. Each drop of your colostrum contains around seven million infection-fighting white blood cells, more than double that found in mature breast milk. This is just one reason why it's fitting that in ancient writings mothers' milk was known as white blood.

Mother's milk is also power-packed with germ-killing proteins called immunoglobulins. Immunoglobulin A (IgA) coats the lining of baby's immature intestines like a protective paint, helping prevent germs from leaking through. Amazingly, preterm milk is twice as rich in IgA as term milk. Mother's milk also accelerates the development of baby's own immune system. Studies show that blood levels of immunoglobulins manufactured by baby are higher in breastfed babies.

The immune profile of your milk is updated continually. Mother's body makes the antibodies her baby needs. When mothers and preemies enjoy skin-to-skin contact during kangaroo care, they share germs. Then mother's mature immune system develops antibodies to the hospital germs to which baby is exposed. These immunities appear in mother's milk and help baby combat infection. Mother's milk comes to the rescue and makes up for baby's inability to respond quickly to germs.

All these infection-fighting substances in mother's milk make a big difference to baby's health. One study showed that the infection rate among nonbreastfed preemies was over twice that of preemies who received their mother's milk. Numerous studies of full-term infants show lower rates of respiratory infections, ear infections, and gastrointestinal illnesses in babies who are breastfed. Consider your milk your baby's first immunization against disease.

Helps digestion. Preemies need to do a lot of growing — fast! Yet, their immature intestines may have a hard time processing

---

SCIENCE SAYS:
MORE MILK FROM MOTHER =
LESS INFECTION IN BABY

Preemies are prone to infections. In recent studies, sepsis, a serious infection in baby's bloodstream, occurred twice as often in formula-fed preemies as in preemies who received breast milk.

---

feedings. Mother's milk acts as a dose of "internal medicine." It contains a special substance called epidermal growth factor (EGF), which stimulates the growth of the cells lining baby's intestines, making them better able to digest food. Preterm milk is slightly higher in EGF than term milk is just when your baby needs it — in the early weeks right after birth. Because breast milk helps the intestines mature faster, breastfed babies are less likely to experience milk intolerances or food allergies.

Breast milk is appropriately dubbed the easy in/easy out food. It is easier to digest at the upper end and makes softer stools that are easier to pass at the lower end. Again, this is especially important for preemies. The immature lining of a preemie's intestines is unable to produce enough enzymes for optimal digestion, especially for the digestion of fat, the prime source of the calories needed for growth. You guessed it! Mother's milk comes to the rescue with large amounts of lipase, the enzyme needed to break down milk fat in the intestines. It also provides other enzymes that speed the digestion of proteins and carbohydrates. Premature intestines have decreased lactase — the enzyme that digests the main carbohydrate, lactose.

Breast milk contains lactase to help this temporary deficiency. Approximately 90 percent of human milk is digested and absorbed by baby, compared with only 60 percent of infant formula.

Maintains a well-balanced system.

Some vitamins and minerals in breast milk are present in relatively small amounts but enjoy a high level of bioavailability, which means a greater percentage of these nutrients is absorbed by baby compared with the vitamins and minerals in formulas. Better bioavailability also means baby's intestines don't have to work as hard to digest the milk. Baby can, therefore, divert this saved energy into growing.

Dr. Alan Lucas, a leading neonatal researcher, believes that a lack of appropriate nutrition during early life can have a permanent effect on how the body grows and functions overall.

Reduces the risk of reflux. Not only is mother's milk better digested, but less of it is spit up. Preemies are at greater risk for gastroesophageal reflux disease (GERD). Normally, a band of muscle where the esophagus joins the stomach contracts after feeding, acting like a valve to prevent milk and stomach contents from regurgitating back up into the esophagus. This muscle is immature in preemies, so they spit up more frequently. This regurgitation can be painful, because stomach acids irritate the lining of the esophagus, producing a condition something like heartburn. GERD happens less often in breastfed babies, primarily because breast milk is digested quickly and empties from the stomach twice as fast as formula does. Less reflux may be one reason why breastfed babies enjoy more peaceful sleep. (For more on gastroesophageal reflux disease, see page 195.)

Prevents necrotizing enterocolitis (NEC). This severe inflammatory bowel condition (see page 198) is one of the most serious, and sometimes fatal, complications of preterm birth. It occurs in 2 to 5 percent of preemies. In a large study of nearly one thousand preemies, the incidence of NEC was six to ten times greater in infants who were exclusively formula-fed than in those who received human milk exclusively. The incidence of NEC was three times greater in preemies who received human milk plus formula than in the exclusively human milk–fed group. Among preemies over 30 weeks of age, formula-fed infants were twenty times more likely to develop NEC than human milk–fed infants were.

Promotes better breathing. Breathing problems are the most common medical

---

SCIENCE SAYS:
BREAST MILK–FED PREEMIES SHOW FASTER FEEDING PROGRESS

One study showed that breast milk–fed preemies reached full tube feedings by eight days of age, compared with twelve days for formula-fed, and began oral feeds by twenty-two days, compared with thirty-one days for formula-fed preemies. In another study, breast milk–fed preemies required an average of ten fewer days of IV nutrition than did the formula-fed preemies.

concern with premature infants, mainly because of the immaturity of the airways and air sacs involved in breathing (see Respiratory Distress Syndrome, page 183). Again, enter mother's milk as medicine. The growth factors mentioned above may help lung tissue mature faster.

Premature babies find it easier to coordinate sucking, swallowing, and breathing during breastfeeding than they do during bottlefeeding. Once upon a time, it was assumed that breastfeeding was more work, and therefore more stressful for a preemie. For this reason, it used to be customary in special care nurseries to initiate bottlefeeding before allowing a baby to breastfeed. Newer studies have shown just the opposite to be true. Infants have more stable heart and respiratory rates, higher blood oxygen levels, and fewer episodes of apnea and bradycardia (low breathing and heart rates) while feeding at the breast. The reason for this seems to be that breastfed babies have a better suck-breathe pattern. Baby is better able to control the flow of milk from the breast than from the bottle, since milk from the breast will not flow unless baby is actively sucking. Breastfed babies have been shown to have more rhythmic sucking patterns. They suck in bursts and pauses and know just when to rest and when to suck so that they'll get the most milk with the least amount of effort. Energy saved during feedings can be used to grow. One research study demonstrated that young preemies breathe while they suck (but not swallow) at the breast, but they don't breathe while sucking on a bottle. As another pulmonary perk, if breast milk does go down the wrong way during a feeding, it will not irritate baby's lungs as much as aspirated formula can.

> ### SCIENCE SAYS: BREASTFEEDING PREEMIES ENJOY HIGHER BLOOD OXYGEN LEVELS
>
> Studies show that preemies have better breathing coordination and higher blood oxygen levels during breastfeeding compared with bottlefeeding preemies.

Builds better bones. Preemies tend to have lower bone mineral content, which can lead to slower bone growth. Compared with formula-fed infants, breastfed preemies at five years of age have a higher bone mineralization.

Builds healthier skin. The thinner, underdeveloped skin of a premature infant is more prone to irritation than that of a term baby. In our pediatric practice, we have noticed that the skin of breastfed preemies is less dry and scaly, and these babies have less eczema. This may be epidermal growth factor at work, or it may be the result of the healthier fats in breast milk. In the final month of pregnancy, a baby lays down a lot of fat beneath the thin skin. Preemies miss out on this development and need the nutritious fats in your milk for healthy skin.

As you can see, your milk helps your preemie grow better from head to toe. And the long-term benefits of breastfeeding make it a wise investment in the future health of your infant. The incidence of just about every disease from diabetes to SIDS is lower in the breastfed infant.

IF YOU ARE UNDECIDED ABOUT WHETHER OR NOT TO BREASTFEED YOUR PREEMIE . . .

To help you make a final decision, we ask you to go through the following steps:

Read all about it. Read about the unique benefits of human milk for preemies (see page 83). In our opinion, human milk should be considered necessary, not optional, for preemies. Read about how, besides being best for baby, breastfeeding is also good for you. (See below.)

Consider the alternative. Although you are unlikely to read this statement in any other book, it is scientifically correct: *Commercially available infant formulas are simply not as good for premature babies as breast milk is.*

Surprised? Look at it this way: With breast milk, preemies get more for less: more nutrition with less expenditure of energy. Nutrients in breast milk have a higher level of bioavailability, which means baby can use a high proportion of these nutrients and there is less waste for the intestines to process. With formula, the manufacturers have to add larger amounts of each nutrient to make sure that an adequate amount is absorbed into baby's immature intestines and bloodstream. For example, 50 to 75 percent of the important mineral iron is absorbed in breast milk compared with only 4 percent of the iron in formula. So formula companies have to add much more iron to make up for the lower bioavailability. Meanwhile, baby's intestines must work harder to get rid of the excess.

Another benefit of breast milk is the immune protection it offers babies. The various germ-fighting ingredients in human milk guard baby from infection. The friendly proteins in human milk are easy for baby to digest and do not set up allergic reactions. Formula-feeding, on the other hand, exposes baby to foreign proteins from cow's milk or soy. It can cause allergies and offers no protection

WHY BREASTFEEDING IS SO SPECIAL FOR MOTHERS OF PREEMIES

Breastfeeding is also good for mothers, especially mothers of preemies. Not only is a breastfed baby biochemically different, but breastfeeding mothers are biochemically different as well.

It helps mothers cope. Prolactin and oxytocin, the hormones that stimulate a woman's body to make and deliver milk for her baby, also help her cope with stress. Feeding a baby at the breast relaxes a mother. As the feeding progresses, mother mellows and baby drifts peacefully off to sleep — as if both have been given a natural tranquilizer, which is in fact what happens. Mother's milk contains a natural sleep-inducing protein to help relax her baby, and the hormones that are released in mother's body during a feeding give her a sense of calmness and well-being. Even pumping milk for your baby may produce this hormonal effect. While prescription sedatives may have side effects that can impair maternal judgment, the against infection. There are more risks and fewer benefits with formula-feeding.

Instead of deciding right now whether or not you want to tackle the many challenges of breastfeeding your baby, make a decision to simply provide your pumped breast milk for your baby now. It can be given to your baby as soon as she is ready for tube feeding, probably within a few days after birth. You don't even need to make a decision about breastfeeding until your baby is actually ready to feed at the breast.

Give it a "30-day free trial." Even if you had not planned to breastfeed (for whatever reasons), we suggest you commit yourself to a 30-day free trial of pumping breast milk for your preemie. Your breasts are going to make milk in the first week after birth anyway, whether you want them to or not. Why let such precious medicine go to waste? Unless there is a medical reason that prevents you from providing breast milk for your baby, please give your baby

your milk at least during the first month. This critical time is when your preemie needs it most. After the first month, you can reassess your feeding choice and use the regimen that works best for you and your baby.

In our experience, having a preemie has often changed a mother's mind about breastfeeding. Once you see the effects on your baby — and yourself — you may want to continue. Don't even think about whether you want to breastfeed for months (or even years). Take it a week at a time. Save the long-term decisions about feeding for later.

Suppose during the first week or so you decided not to breastfeed but now you've changed your mind. Can you start now? Yes! Or perhaps you were ill and not able to begin pumping immediately. You can still breastfeed. With a high dose of commitment and the help of a professional lactation consultant, you can relactate to get your body to produce milk to give your baby.

hormones from breastfeeding can actually promote relaxed, intuitive mothering.

It helps mothers feel connected. During the days and weeks that a premature baby needs special care, pumping milk and breastfeeding may be the only things that a mother can do for her baby, and they are things that *only* she can do. Premature birth disrupts nature's plan for keeping mother and baby connected. Expressing milk and eventually breastfeeding nourish the physical and psychological bond begun during pregnancy. This helps

you get connected with your baby, despite the medical circumstances that can keep you apart. The transition from being a working professional and master of your fate to being the mother of a premature baby, or even a full-term baby, is a profound one, particularly in the first six months. Breastfeeding gives you an opportunity to reflect in a quiet, private place on your life and your hopes and expectations of being a mother. It makes the physiological connection emotional as well. These are not easy ideas for new moms to consider when they are overwhelmed with worry and stress, but try to find the time. Breastfeeding, pumping, or merely sitting by the side of your baby can provide that time for you.

I was very determined to succeed, because that was one thing I could do for my baby that no other person could. It made me feel like I was really a mommy.

◆

The nurse was so encouraging. She made me feel like my body might actually be getting something right! This was a boost, since I was just getting over my guilt from not being able to carry him to term.

It helps mothers get to know their babies. Pumping milk keeps you involved in your baby's daily care. The more involved you are, the better you will know your baby. After a few weeks of this bedside maternal nursing, you'll be amazed at how much effect your observations will have on the overall management of your baby's care.

When your baby is ready to nurse at the breast, breastfeeding becomes an exercise in baby-reading. It increases your sensitivity to any changes in your baby. As you learn to judge whether baby is feeding effectively and when it's time to take a break or switch sides, you are learning to understand your baby's cues. Your responsiveness to what baby needs plays an important role in her development.

Dr. Bill notes: During my thirty years as a mother-and-baby watcher, I have been impressed by the increased sensitivity breastfeeding mothers have toward subtle changes in their babies.

It helps mothers be healthier. Breastfeeding helps you lose your pregnancy weight faster and decreases your risk of breast and ovarian cancer and osteoporosis.

Now that you understand why you and your milk are so important to your baby, here's how to get the best start.

HOW BREASTFEEDING WORKS

The birth of a baby and the delivery of the placenta that follows trigger hormonal changes in a mother's body that lead to the production of milk. Milk production follows pregnancy, regardless of whether the baby is born at term or many weeks ahead of schedule. In other words, your body will make milk after your baby's delivery whether you want it to or not.

At first, the breasts produce a substance called colostrum, a kind of early milk. It is yellowish in color and sticky and available only in small amounts in the first days after birth. Yet it is packed with immunities and other substances that make it the perfect first feeding for immature tummies. After two or three days (sometimes longer), milk production goes into full swing, when your milk "comes in." Your breasts fill up and swell with milk, more milk than even a full-term baby may know what to do with.

The next part of the process is crucial: the milk must be removed from the breasts so that mother's body knows it should continue to make more. When baby nurses often over the next several weeks, mother's milk production adapts to match the amount of milk baby is taking. Her supply meets baby's demand. As baby grows and requires more milk, mother's breasts respond to baby's sucking by increasing their output.

What happens when baby cannot breastfeed. The baby's role in milk production is very important. If the milk is not removed from the breasts, they will stop making milk. Substances in the milk itself and sensors in the breast signal the body to shut down milk production, since the milk doesn't seem to be needed.

So what happens when a baby, because of sickness or prematurity, is unable to nurse? Even if baby is not yet ready for milk feedings, he will need the milk someday. Enter the breast pump, a substitute for the nursing baby. Pumping solves two problems:

- It gets milk out of the breasts for a baby who is not yet strong enough to do so by himself.
- It stimulates the breasts to continue to produce milk, so that the milk will be there when the baby is ready to nurse.

PUMPING MILK FOR YOUR PREEMIE

If your preemie is too young or too sick to nurse directly from your breast, you will need to express your milk with a breast pump. While "nursing" from a mechanical pump is not the warm and maternal experience you may have envisioned, pumping your breasts soon after birth has the following benefits:

- It gets you immediately involved in the care of your preemie.

- It gets your "supermilk," colostrum, flowing.
- It stimulates maternal and relaxing hormones that help you mother and cope.
- It builds your milk bank with this "liquid gold" for later use.

Pumping your breasts not only provides milk for your baby, but it also tells your body not to quit lactating. Frequent pumping is especially important during the first two to three weeks after birth. It "primes the pump" by activating more prolactin receptor cells in the breast. This sets you up for a better milk supply and more efficient milk making in the months to come.

Pumping may seem like a strange process, especially at first. But in the long run, pumping will make it possible for you and your baby to enjoy the pleasures and benefits of breastfeeding for many months to come. Keep these long-term goals in mind. Here are nine tips for pumping for your preemie:

1. Pick the Right Pump

Your special care nursery should provide you with a hospital-grade pump with a dual collection system. This type of pump has three major benefits:

- Efficiency. You can pump more milk in less time.
- Gentleness. It will not traumatize sensitive breast tissue.
- Effectiveness. Double-pumping (i.e., pumping both breasts at the same time) stimulates the body to produce more milk and higher levels of prolactin, the milk-making hormone.

Read the detailed instructions that come with the pump several times, even after someone shows you how to use the pump. It may be hard for you to take in this information in the first few days after your baby's birth, when there is so much to learn and worry about. Ask your partner or a friend with breast pump experience to help you.

2. Consult a Lactation Specialist

The neonatal nurse or lactation consultant at the hospital will show you how to put your pump parts together and how to use the pump. The lactation consultant will become a very important person to you during your baby's hospital stay. Get to know her well, as she will be a valuable source of information and support during the time you are pumping and when your baby is ready to feed at the breast.

3. Prepare Your Surroundings

While you are still in the hospital, ask to have a breast pump in your room. You will also need a pump at home; the nurses or lactation consultant can arrange for you to rent one. Some hospitals have a designated private pumping room near the NICU, in which there are pumps, comfortable chairs, and a sink for you to use. In the first few days, as you are getting used to pumping your milk, you may want to pump mostly in the pumping room. Later on, many mothers find they can pump more effectively at baby's bedside.

I was able to pump more milk while at the bedside of my baby, looking at her while I pumped. I would picture her soon replacing the pump at my breast. That *gave my milk a boost. It was much better than trying to express milk in the pumping room.*

You will need a comfortable chair and a table next to it to hold the pump and the containers for the milk. Wash your hands thoroughly before you begin, including under your fingernails. Assemble the pump parts and arrange your clothing so that you can pump both breasts at once. If you're pumping at your baby's bedside, you'll probably want to close the curtains to ensure your privacy.

4. Prepare Your Mind and Body

Besides preparing your surroundings, prepare your mind and body. Expressing milk is more than a mechanical encounter between your breasts and a pump. Take a few minutes to relax before you start to pump. Close your eyes and exhale and inhale deeply. Visualize a flowing stream or a quiet forest. Even better, visualize your baby nursing and your milk freely flowing. Relax your mind so that your body is free to respond to the pump. Some mothers find it helps to "prime the pump" by drinking a couple glasses of water right before pumping. Breast massage, working from the chest wall down to the nipple, can also get the milk flowing. (See Perking Up Your Milk Supply, page 99, for instructions on how to massage your breasts, or ask a lactation consultant for help.)

5. Start Pumping

Now that you've gotten your mind and body set, it's time to go. Set the pump at its gentlest suction setting. Center your

LOVING AND HATING YOUR BREAST PUMP

On the one hand, your breast pump makes it possible for you to give your baby the nutrition designed by nature to help her grow and thrive. On the other hand, that cycling, suctioning, heavy machine, with its cold plastic tubes and funnels, is anything but natural. Many a mother has experienced a love/hate relationship with her breast pump. As with any other difficult relationship, a sense of humor helps keep things in perspective.

You may even develop close ties to your pump. Your body may become so conditioned to pumping that just looking at the pump triggers your milk to let down. Some mothers find that their milk lets down easily when they pump, but not so quickly when they finally feed their babies at the breast. The milk-ejection reflex (MER) is conditioned to the pumping ritual; it takes several feeding sessions to recondition the MER to feeding baby. Skin-to-skin contact in kangaroo care speeds this transition.

Success Stories — What the Experts Say

Enjoy these bits of advice from pumping mothers of preemies:

I was determined to give my twins my milk, so I pumped every three hours, including at nighttime so that I would produce enough milk for both babies. I'm so happy I was able to do that for them. It was worth the extra effort.

◆

Be sure a lactation consultant sees you right away in the NICU to help you get started with pumping tips.

◆

Pump right away after birth, so your baby can get your power-packed colostrum.

◆

The medical staff were great. They really encouraged me to continue pumping, and when I was having trouble, they were my cheering section.

◆

Be sure you have two hospital-grade pumps — one at home and one at the hospital.

nipple in the pump's flange. You may feel less awkward if you pump only one breast at a time at first, using the single-collecting setup. Move on to double pumping as you feel more confident. If the pump comes with more than one size flange, choose the one that best fits your breast — big enough that your nipple and areola do not rub against the sides of the flange but a close enough fit to stimulate the breast effectively. You may want to experiment with different flanges to see which one works best for you.

Turn the pump on. You will see your nipple and areola move back and forth in the flange as the pump goes through its suction-and-release cycle. In the first few days after birth, you will be able to collect only a teaspoon or so of colostrum at each pumping session. After your milk comes in, you will notice that a minute or two of pumping triggers your milk-ejection reflex (MER), or letdown, and milk will spray from your nipple into the flange and then drain into the collection bottle. Increasing the suction setting on the pump may help the milk to flow more quickly, but don't set the suction so high that pumping becomes uncomfortable. Suction that is too strong will make your nipples sore. Remember, pumping should not hurt, as pain may inhibit your MER and you'll pump less milk.

Prime the pumps. Before you begin each pumping session, gently massage the areola and nipple of each breast. This may help stimulate your milk letdown better than pumping alone. Massaging the entire breast (see below) may also enhance your milk letdown.

Massage your breasts periodically after pumping. In order to ensure you are completely draining each breast, massage your breasts with your fingertips starting at the outer edge and moving in a circular pattern around your breast and spiraling inward. If you feel any lumps along the way, gently massage that area inward toward your nipple to drain what is probably a plugged duct filled with milk.

6. How Long Should You Pump?

Continue pumping until your milk is no longer flowing, and then pump two minutes longer. The extra pumping may trigger an additional MER and produce more milk. Once your milk has come in, expect to spend about ten or fifteen minutes pumping each breast at each pumping session. (Pumping both breasts simultaneously saves time and also yields higher blood prolactin levels and more milk.)

Don't pump for longer than thirty minutes. Longer periods of pumping could make you sore and really don't do much to boost your milk supply. Shorter, more frequent pumping sessions are more effective at increasing milk production.

The fat content of your milk increases during a feeding or pumping session. This means that the milk pumped at the end of the expression period, after you have experienced the MER one or more times, is higher in calories than the first milk you pump. We call this the "grow milk," because it is important to your baby's weight gain. This is why it's important to pump until you can't get any more milk from the breast.

7. How Often to Pump

Pumping should mimic the feeding behavior of a newborn during the early weeks, and newborns feed frequently. Plan on pumping every two to three hours during the day for a total of eight to ten pumping sessions in each twenty-four-hour period. Your body makes more milk in the morning, so you may want to pump more often in the morning and early afternoon. It's best to have the same kind of hospital-grade breast pump at home. Set your alarm so that you can wake up and pump at least once a night, about four hours after you go to bed. Frequent pumping in the early weeks helps establish a good milk supply for the long term.

After three weeks of this frequent pumping schedule, you may be able to maintain a good milk supply while cutting back slightly on the time you spend with your breast pump. If you can, though, stick with the frequent pumping. When you have an abundant milk supply, your milk flows more quickly and baby does not have to work as hard while nursing. This helps get more milk into baby during her early feedings at the breast.

8. How Much Milk Will You Pump?

During the first few days, you may be able to pump only a teaspoonful of colostrum at a time. While small in volume, colostrum is rich in nutrients and contains high concentrations of antibodies, infection fighters, and other substances that prepare the lining of baby's stomach for the feedings to come. Mothers of preemies often produce more colostrum and continue to produce it for a few days more. Be sure to save every precious drop and ask that your colostrum be given to your baby at his very first feeding, either orally or by tube.

If your baby is ready for milk feedings but not for nipple feedings, your milk will be given to him through a tube that goes from his mouth or nose into his stomach. This is called gavage feeding. Very little milk adheres to the sides of the tubing, so you don't have to worry about your precious milk going to waste. Since colostrum is thicker and stickier than mature milk, the nurse may dilute it with sterile water to make it easier to give your baby.

You will notice that your milk becomes much more plentiful after a few days of pumping. This early milk is a beautiful golden white color because of the colostrum that is mixed through it. Again, it is important to save this "white gold" for your baby because of the high concentrations of antibodies and growth hormones. Due to the stress of a preterm delivery and, perhaps, medical complications such as a cesarean, mothers of preemies often take longer to progress from pumping a few drops to an ounce or more at each pumping. Think positively and continue to pump often. If your breasts are feeling swollen and engorged, frequent pumping will bring relief.

By ten days or so after the birth, you'll probably be producing 20 ounces (600 ml) or more of milk each day. In fact, many mothers of preemies eventually produce more milk than their baby needs in the early weeks. Building up an abundant milk supply in the early weeks ensures that your body will continue to produce milk efficiently in the weeks to come. If you find that you are pumping less than 12 ounces (350 ml) per day by 2 weeks postpartum, this may mean that you are not establishing an abundant supply to meet baby's growing needs in the months to come. We strongly suggest you take steps now to increase your supply. This is much more easily done sooner rather than later. (See Perking Up Your Milk Supply, page 99.)

Your milk will gradually change from its golden color and become white with a bluish tinge. When the milk sits in a container undisturbed, it separates into layers and the cream rises to the top. (Milk fresh from your breasts does not undergo homogenization like the cow's milk at the supermarket.) You might think that this milk looks thinner or weaker than the early milk, but rest assured, it is still full of the proteins, vitamins, and fats that your baby needs, along with all the special immune properties that make breast milk so good for premature babies.

Because very premature infants require greater amounts of some nutrients than mother's milk can provide, the milk is sometimes mixed with a powdered or liquid human milk fortifier before it is given to baby. Don't interpret this as meaning that your milk is not good enough for your baby. Your doctor may recommend that your baby receive these extra nutrients temporarily. (See Human Milk Fortifier — Boosting Your Breast Milk, right.)

9. Store Your "Liquid Gold"

You want to preserve and protect your precious milk. How you store your milk affects how well its immune properties are preserved. Another storage concern is protecting the milk (and therefore, your baby) from bacteria growth.

You need to label the milk carefully and make appropriate decisions about freezing it or storing it in the refrigerator. Your hospital may supply containers and preprinted labels for you to use when storing your milk. Your hospital may also have specific procedures for you to follow when pumping and transporting milk for your preemie. Follow these carefully.

The milk you pump during the first half of a pumping session (called foremilk) is lower in fat, whereas the hindmilk pumped in the second half of a session has a higher fat content. It even looks thicker and more white. You may choose to store some hindmilk in separate bottles to have on hand in case baby needs some higher-calorie milk for a period of fast catch-up growth.

Containers. Some hospital nurseries prefer that you use glass containers; others prefer plastic. Breast pump manufacturers sell special plastic bags that can be used to store breast milk, and in some cases,

---

HUMAN MILK FORTIFIER — BOOSTING YOUR BREAST MILK

While breast milk is by far the best food for your baby, it is often necessary to add human milk fortifier (HMF) to increase the overall calories, especially if baby is born weighing less than 3½ pounds (1500 grams). HMF contains certain vitamins, minerals, and protein to help ensure baby is getting adequate amounts. Interestingly, the protein content of breast milk decreases dramatically in the first few weeks. But we also know that protein is crucial for weight gain and growth. So the question is, are preemies supposed to be fed less protein, because this is what happens naturally in breast milk? Or should we fortify baby's feeds to make up for this decrease in protein? Most experts feel HMF is beneficial for preemies. If your doctor advises that this be added to your breast milk, don't take it as a criticism of the value of your milk. The doctor simply wants your baby to get a little added protein for growth. HMF should be added to breast milk right before feeding. Breast milk with added HMF should not be stored, as this can cause contamination with bacteria.

---

these can be attached directly to the pump so that the milk flows right into the bag. Each type of container has its advantages.

Glass containers and hard-sided plastic containers protect the milk well and sit directly on a shelf in the freezer or refrigerator. It is easy for nurses to pour the milk from these containers into whatever

PERKING UP YOUR MILK SUPPLY

If your milk supply is dwindling, you can take steps to build it up again. Here are some suggestions:

- Pump more often — every two hours during the day, at least once during the night.
- Massage your breasts before and during pumping sessions to stimulate your MER and move milk down toward the nipple. After applying a warm towel or a cloth diaper soaked in warm water to your breasts, use your fingertips to stroke from the top of the breast down over the nipple, using a light feather touch. Then, using a motion similar to the one you use when doing a monthly breast exam, massage the milk-producing glands by pressing the breast firmly into the chest with the flat of your fingers. Begin at the top of the breast and work in a spiral motion around the breast down toward the areola.
- Set up a "nursing station," a special place at home for pumping, with a comfortable chair, snacks, and all your equipment, plus books or puzzles for a toddler or older child. Follow the same routine every time you pump. This conditions your milk-ejection reflex.
- Pump at the hospital immediately after visiting your baby or holding your baby.
- Pump at your baby's bedside. Ask the nurses to set up a screen so that you can have some privacy. Look at your baby while you pump.
- When not at your baby's bedside, think about your baby while pumping. Look at a picture or cuddle a piece of clothing or his blanket against your cheek.
- Another approach is to think about something else while pumping. Some mothers release more milk if they visualize rivers flowing through the forest or a peaceful ocean beach. Escape in your mind from the tensions of having a premature baby. Wear headphones and listen to a special tape or CD.
- Check your pump. Parts and seals do wear out, making the pump less effective. Call the pump manufacturer for information, or talk to the lactation consultant who supplied you with the pump.
- If you are not using a hospital-grade electric breast pump, move up to this luxury pump. It makes a difference.
- Use a double-sided pump. Frequent stimulation to both breasts will increase your milk supply.
- Ask your lactation consultant about taking a galactogogue — herbs, teas, or medications that may stimulate your milk supply. There are no scientific, controlled studies supporting the use of herbs such as fenugreek or fennel to increase milk supply, but some mothers and lactation consultants believe they make a difference.
- Sometimes prescription drugs are used to increase a mother's milk supply. Metoclopramide, 10 milligrams one to three times a day for seven to ten days, has been shown to increase milk supply and raise prolactin levels. If the neonatal staff is unfamiliar with this treatment, discuss it with your own doctor or with the hospital lactation consultant.

type of setup is being used to feed your baby. However, research has shown that breast milk leukocytes (white blood cells important to immune functions) stick to the sides of glass containers and stay behind when the milk is poured out. On the other hand, research has also shown that milk stored in glass containers has a higher number of leukocytes, which suggests that over time, the leukocytes that stick to the glass are released back into the milk. If your pumped milk is to be given to your baby immediately, it may be best to avoid glass containers.

The plastic bags that are designed specifically to store breast milk are made of polyethylene, and they are thicker and heavier than the plastic nurser bags used with disposable baby bottles. These bags come with secure closures and do a good job of protecting the nutrients and immunities in the milk. For easier handling, you'll want to place them inside another container in your refrigerator or freezer. If your pump allows you to pump milk directly into the sterile bag, you minimize the chances of your milk picking up bacteria from the container or your hands. However, some experts believe plastic bags are more easily contaminated than hard containers. Consult your NICU staff for recommendations.

Labeling. Every container should be labeled with your baby's name and the date and time the milk was collected. If you are taking any medications, this information should also be written on the label. Check with your baby's nurses about other information needed on the label, such as your baby's hospital ID number. The nurses may be able to give you a sheet of labels preprinted with your baby's name and ID to which you can add information about the milk. It's important to make a note of which containers hold your colostrum (e.g., Day 1, 2, 3, etc.), since you want your baby to get this power-packed milk first. Colostrum can be refrigerated for up to forty-eight hours; beyond that, it should be frozen.

Freeze, refrigerate, or feed fresh?

Freezing destroys some of the live cells in human milk and deactivates hormones and enzymes that aid in digestion and promote baby's growth. Refrigerated breast milk is better, and fresh milk is best of all. Frozen breast milk is still very, very good for your baby and far superior to infant formula. Because fresh breast milk preserves more anti-infection substances, try to give your baby your fresh, unfrozen milk whenever possible. However, for younger preemies who don't start tube feedings until they are a few weeks old, it's important you use your frozen colostrum first, then the milk that you pumped during that first week. This first milk, even frozen, is better for baby's immature intestines than your more mature fresh milk is. Once baby seems to be tolerating feedings well, you can skip some of your frozen stores and start giving baby your fresh milk.

Studies show that human milk does not show any significant bacterial growth when kept at room temperature (66 to 72° F, or 19 to 22° C) for ten hours or in the refrigerator for up to eight days. However, guidelines for storing milk for preemies are usually more conservative, since preemies are more vulnerable to bacterial infections and are dependent on expressed milk for long periods of time. It is wise to be cautious.

The hospital staff can give you specific instructions about storing your milk so that they can use it efficiently and in a timely fashion. Here are some general guidelines:

- If you pump during the time you are visiting your baby at the hospital, the nurses may be able to give him your milk fresh and still warm.
- If the milk will be given to baby in the next twenty-four to forty-eight hours, store it in the refrigerator immediately. Milk not used within forty-eight hours can be transferred to the freezer for longer storage.
- It's best to use a separate container for each pumping session, although you may wish to combine very small amounts of milk in a single container later.
- If your baby is not ready for milk feedings yet, freeze the milk right after it's pumped so that it can be given to your baby later. Some hospitals give the oldest-pumped milk to baby first, so that baby receives colostrum, then transitional milk, just like at the breast. Pay attention to which milk the nurses are using to be sure your baby gets your milk in the right order.
- Human milk can be kept safely for three to four months in your refrigerator's separate freezer compartment. It can be stored in a deep freezer for at least six months. You will be glad to have milk "banked" in the freezer if baby's demand gets ahead of what you are able to pump in the weeks to come.
- Bring refrigerated or frozen milk to the hospital packed in a cooler filled with ice or "blue ice" packs.

Amounts. Nobody likes to see precious breast milk go down the drain. But hospitals have different policies about what to do with the milk left in the container after baby has been fed. Some save human milk in the refrigerator for the next feeding. Others, concerned about bacterial growth, dump it. Ask the nurses how much milk to store in each container so that waste is kept to a minimum.

Medications in mother's milk. Tell your baby's doctors if you are taking any kind of medication during the time you are pumping milk or breastfeeding your premature baby. Information about any medication you are taking should be included on the label of the milk you pump. While most medications are compatible with breastfeeding, premature infants have greater difficulty breaking down and excreting drugs from their system. If you are taking a medication that could pose problems for your tiny infant, you may have to "pump and dump" your milk for a time, either until you are no longer using the medicine or until your baby is mature enough to handle the small amounts that may appear in your milk.

Managing the dairy. With milk stored both at home and at the hospital, keeping track of the inventory relative to baby's consumption can become challenging. It may help to keep a written log on the refrigerator door at home. Communicate regularly with the nurses. Call before you go to the hospital and find out if you should bring milk from your freezer. If the staff knows that you are coming in to visit and pump, they can schedule baby's feeding so that he receives fresh milk, perhaps even while you are holding him.

Keeping up with the demand. Maintaining a milk supply is not easy. Most mothers of premature babies find that the

BREAST MILK BANKS — FEEDING YOUR BABY DONATED BREAST MILK

In the 1950s and '60s, breast-milk banks were quite popular. Almost all preemies were fed breast milk because preterm infant formulas were not available. When moms couldn't provide breast milk, donor breast milk was used. Then along came HIV and other infectious diseases in the 1980s, and out went the milk banks because of a fear of transmitting these diseases through donated milk. By this time, formula was available, and it was used when Mom couldn't provide breast milk.

Now science is showing how crucial breast milk is for preemies, and more and more moms who can't provide it are turning once again to donated breast milk. Milk banks are available across the United States, but is giving your baby another person's breast milk safe? The answer is yes.

Milk banks operate just like blood banks. They are certified by the Human Milk Banking Association of North America and follow guidelines established by the Centers for Disease Control, the American Academy of Pediatrics, and the Food and Drug Administration (FDA). A mom who donates milk is given an extensive health screening for any risk factors, and blood testing is done to check for infectious diseases. The donated milk is pasteurized (just like cow's milk) and tested to make sure no bacteria or viruses pass into baby.

If you can't provide breast milk to your baby and you want your baby to get donated breast milk instead of formula, you may run into some resistance from the NICU staff. Donated breast milk still has a stigma attached to it in some NICUs because of concern about transmitting infectious diseases. Pasteurizing and processing breast milk causes it to lose some of its nutritional value and live biological factors, so you may hear that it's not worth it. Using bottles of formula is infinitely more convenient than ordering, transporting, and preparing donated breast milk. Donated milk also costs more money up front than formula does. However, research has shown that fears of disease are unfounded and the benefits of even donated breast milk far outweigh the convenience of formula. It has been well proven that donated milk from milk banks does not transmit infectious diseases. Pasteurized donated breast milk with added human milk fortifier (see page 98) has far more nutritional and biological value than formula does. Most enzymes, vitamins, minerals, antibodies, and infection-fighting factors are only slightly reduced or remain unchanged. White blood cells are destroyed, but this actually has an advantage in that it decreases the chance of baby having an allergic reaction to another mom's milk. Moreover, Dr. Nancy Wright's research has shown that the cost savings due to decreased medical problems and shorter hospital stays when donor breast milk is used instead of formula are significant.

We support the use of donor breast milk, and if you want more information on how to obtain it, ask your NICU nursing coordinator. You can also go to www.hmbana.org.

amount of milk they are producing declines as the weeks go by. Your milk supply may also fluctuate with your baby's condition. During a crisis, you may not be able to pump as much. This is normal. With continued pumping, your milk supply will recover. And even if your baby must be supplemented with formula, your milk still provides important benefits. Breastfeeding a premature baby is not an all-or-nothing proposition.

Warming your milk. Never warm your milk in a microwave. This may alter the nutritional content and may warm the milk unevenly, creating hot spots that can harm baby. Place the milk container in a bowl of hot water and warm the milk to body temperature (98° F, or 37° C).

Now you are ready to feed your baby your liquid gold. See chapter 8 for bottle-feeding tips, or see Supplementary Feedings, page 110, for alternatives to the bottle.

HOW TO STOP PUMPING

At some point during baby's early life, you will find that you no longer need to use your breast pump. Perhaps your baby is a few months old and feeding so well at the breast that no more supplemental feedings are needed (in this case, you may have been decreasing your pumping sessions already). Or you may have decided to suddenly discontinue breastfeeding, and you no longer wish to give your baby pumped breast milk. Whatever your situation, when you decide to stop pumping, it is vital that you do so gradually. If you suddenly stop using the pump, you may get painfully engorged with milk, which may lead to mastitis, an infection inside the breasts. You can prevent this by dropping one pumping session every two or three days. For example, if you have been pumping eight times a day, then it should take you two to three weeks to wean yourself off the breast pump. If your situation does not allow you such a gradual weaning process, you can use this faster method: Pump for a few minutes several times a day whenever your breasts begin to feel uncomfortably full. Pump only enough milk to ease the fullness. Your milk production will slow down and stop within several days. This accelerated process, however, increases your risk of mastitis. Symptoms of mastitis include large, painful lumps inside the breasts, flulike symptoms, and fevers, if the inflammation is advanced.

Feeding Your Preemie at the Breast

THROUGH ALL THE UPS AND downs of pumping, mothers of preemies look forward to that big maternal moment when baby can begin breastfeeding. Making the transition from pumping and gavage feeding to feeding your baby at the breast can be challenging. You will need plenty of "P&P" — patience and persistence — as you help your baby discover and refine his sucking skills.

WHEN CAN YOU START?

The age and stage at which a premature baby is ready to begin feeding at the breast is a preemie-by-preemie decision. Each nursery has its own criteria. Some specify that baby must be a certain weight or gestational age. Other very pro-breastfeeding nurseries encourage mothers to begin feedings at the breast once the baby is no longer in need of ventilator breathing assistance and can maintain a reasonably stable body temperature outside the isolette for short periods of time. This will be around 30 to 32 weeks' gestational age for many preemies but may be as young as 28 weeks for some.

One study showed that even extremely low-birth-weight babies (less than 1½ pounds) can safely latch onto the breast. Another study showed that preemies can safely latch onto the breast as early as 28 weeks, can efficiently obtain milk from the breast around 31 weeks, and can achieve full exclusive breastfeeding by 36 weeks.

"GET ACQUAINTED WITH THE BREAST" FEEDINGS

Remember, your baby's sucking skills are immature, her mouth is small, and she tires easily. So, the first feedings will introduce her to the breast, not fill her up with milk. This is why we call these early feedings "taste" feedings. "Drink" feedings will come later.

Your baby's first feedings may actually occur during kangaroo care, which is a kind of prelude to breastfeeding. Babies who are held skin-to-skin against Mother's chest often seek her nipple. Neonatal researchers have observed that babies as young as 28 weeks are able to root and grasp the nipple. Rooting is an instinctual behavior in which a baby opens her mouth wide and turns her head, searching for the breast. Babies in kangaroo care may wriggle into a position where they can lick, nuzzle, or even latch on.

This is a time to introduce baby to your breast, and your breast to baby, with no particular feeding goals in mind. If you empty your breast by pumping right before kangaroo care, baby can enjoy the taste and smell of a small amount of your milk without being overwhelmed by the flow. Expect your baby to just nuzzle and suck for a brief period of time before getting tired and drifting off to sleep. Enjoy just sitting and relaxing with your baby nestled against your breast. When baby awakens, let him try again if he wants to. A few "just for practice" sessions like this will prepare him for more serious breastfeeding soon.

FIRST LATCH-ON FEEDINGS

Expect first attempts at breastfeeding to be awkward for both you and baby. Learning to breastfeed is a process. Your breastfeeding relationship with your preemie won't be built in a day. Along with the times when you feel happy that your baby is finally nursing, there will be times when you feel frustrated by the whole process. You need patience, persistence, and, ideally, another pair of hands to get you started.

What you should know about baby's behavior at the breast. Sucking vigorously enough to get milk from the breast is hard work for preemies. Because their sucking skills are not thoroughly developed, they may expend a lot of energy in oral feedings and in learning when to suck and when to breathe. This is why tiny preemies who are stressed by medical problems do not receive oral feedings until they are older and stronger. Yet, as we have mentioned earlier, breastfeeding is significantly less stressful for preemies than bottlefeeding, and many preemies are being put to the breast earlier than previously. Since babies lose most of their body heat through their heads, remember to keep your baby's "preemie cap" on during early feedings.

During these first practice feedings, you will notice that your baby exhibits two types of sucking: nonnutritive sucking (NNS) and nutritive sucking (NS). With NNS, baby may lick and suck in short bursts and pauses but not suck with enough vigor and suction to obtain much milk. This is the kind of sucking you will see during kangaroo care. NNS relaxes baby. It also facilitates milk digestion by stimulating the flow of saliva, which is rich in digestive enzymes. If you express a few drops of milk, your baby can begin taste testing already during this easygoing comfort sucking.

With nutritive sucking, baby latches onto the whole nipple and part of the areola and coordinates sucking with swallowing and breathing. Nutritive sucking uses the motion of the entire lower jaw along with a wavelike action of the tongue to extract milk from the breast, at a rate of approximately one suck per second. Baby swallows milk after every one or two sucks. In contrast, nonnutritive sucking is faster, uses only the muscles around the mouth, and does not yield much, if any, milk.

Even babies as young as 30 weeks old may show some signs of nutritive sucking, and most preemies will show nutritive sucking at the breast by 32 weeks.

Babies begin a feeding with nonnutritive sucking. The stimulation to the nipple triggers mother's milk-ejection reflex (MER), and as milk begins to flow, baby switches to a more rhythmic, more organized nutritive suck. Nonnutritive sucking may return at the end of the feeding. Lazy, peaceful, nonnutritive sucking calms and soothes babies. If baby's NNS seems more frantic and disorganized, he may be getting tired and may need to stop nursing.

Before you start. Two very important terms in breastfeeding are "positioning" (how you hold your baby) and "latch-on" (how baby takes your breast into his mouth). Proper positioning and latch-on are even more important for preemies than for full-term babies. Preemies have less strength in their jaws and tongue, so it is harder for them to hold the breast in their mouth and create the suction that elongates mother's nipple and draws it back to the place where the soft and hard palate meet. Also, preemies need more head and shoulder support.

Ask for help from the neonatal nurses or lactation specialist at these early feedings. An experienced helper can assist you with getting baby positioned and latched on. She can also help you interpret your baby's cues and behavior at the breast. One or two breastfeeding sessions a day may be all your baby can handle at first. Don't worry about how much milk baby takes in during these first feedings. As your baby becomes more proficient at sucking, he will gradually get more of his food directly from you. Try this sequence:

- *Get comfortable yourself.* Wear clothing that allows easy access to the breast, perhaps a hospital gown that opens in the front. Ask for a comfortable chair and close the privacy screen. Use pillows behind your back and shoulders, under your elbow, and in your lap to support baby's body and your own. A footstool is a must!
- *Partially empty your breasts.* If you find your milk flows too fast, empty your breasts by pumping right before the first feeding so baby can enjoy the taste and smell of a small amount of your milk without being overwhelmed by the flow. If your breasts are very full, express enough milk to soften the nipple and areola so that it is easier for baby to grasp the breast. To encourage baby to want to suck from your nipple, hand express a few drops that she can enjoy licking from your nipple.

Try different positions. Because preemies need a lot of back and neck support while nursing, the traditional cradle hold, where the baby is brought to the breast with his head resting in the crook of the mother's elbow, may not work well at first. Instead, try one of the following:

- *Reverse cradle hold.* Start out by holding baby with his head in the crook of your elbow, his body extending across yours, along your arm. Then switch hands. So, if you are preparing to nurse with your left breast, your right hand will support baby's upper back and neck. Use your left hand to support your breast.
- *Clutch hold.* When you are nursing at the left breast, support baby's neck and shoulders with your left hand and tuck his body under your left arm. This frees

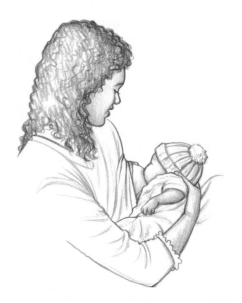

Reverse cradle hold.

your right hand to support your breast. Use pillows at your side to support baby at breast height.

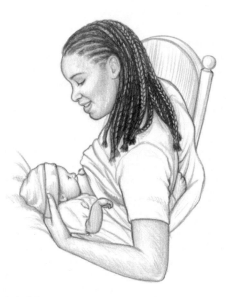

Clutch hold.

In either position, your fingers and thumb will cup the back of baby's neck, from ear to ear. Avoid touching baby's cheeks with your fingers; this can trigger the rooting reflex, causing him to move his head excitedly from side to side. Avoid touching the back of baby's head, too, since this may cause him to arch away from the breast.

Help baby latch on. Support your breast with your hand in the shape of a U or a C, fingers underneath, thumb on top, elbow and wrist in a comfortable position. Then follow these steps to help baby latch on:

- Position baby's nose at the level of your nipple with his head tilted slightly back in the "sniffing" position.
- Brush his lower lip with your nipple to encourage him to open his mouth wide. Ease him onto the breast chin first. Help him to get a good-size mouthful of breast. Keep your fingers out of the way.
- Continue to support baby's shoulders and neck with your hand. Gentle pressure on baby's upper back and neck helps him keep the breast in his mouth and suck longer with less effort.

Once baby is latched on, take a closer look. Baby's tongue should be under the nipple. Baby's lips should be flanged out and his chin pressed into the breast. His nose may or may not be touching the breast. If baby's nose is blocked by breast tissue, pull his body and feet closer to you. This will tilt his head back slightly so that he can breathe more easily. To be sure his lower lip is not puckered inward, try the lower-lip flip: with your index finger, press down gently on baby's chin, which will evert the lower lip for a more efficient latch-on and seal. Or, slip a finger between your breast and baby's mouth to pull the lower lip out. Since it may be difficult for you to bend over and see the position of baby's lower lip, a nurse or your partner can do the lower-lip flip for you. Later on, when baby begins to suck with more pressure, ensuring that baby's lips are turned out rather than puckered will not only help baby nurse more efficiently but also be more comfortable on your nipples.

Many preemies suck only briefly during their first attempts at breastfeeding and soon fall asleep. As preemies get older, they suck longer and in a more organized pattern of nutritive sucking with pauses. If your baby is showing signs of stress or is getting very tired, it's time to end the feeding. Baby may nurse on only one side during these first feedings, so you may want to pump the other breast to keep your supply flowing. When he is bigger and stronger, you can offer the second breast after he has finished nursing on the first side.

Make latch-on easier for baby. Latching on is part instinct, part learned behavior.

Some babies master this skill more easily than others do. Because of baby's weak oral musculature, initially he may be unable to draw much of your areola into his mouth by himself. You need to help him. Remember the cardinal rule for efficient and comfortable latch-on: babies should suck areolas, not just nipples. During the "getting acquainted with the breast" feedings, your preemie may gently suck only your nipple, but eventually you want her to learn to take a good-size mouthful of breast so that her jaws can compress the milk sinuses below the areola. This yields more milk and prevents nipple soreness.

Be patient and persistent while teaching baby to take the breast. If baby has latched onto only the nipple, without taking some of the areola into his mouth, gently break the suction by pressing down on the breast, take him off, and try it again. Here are some techniques to use to get more of your breast into baby's mouth:

• Make a "breast sandwich" that will be easier for baby to grasp. Partially flatten the breast between your thumb and fingers while pushing straight back into the chest wall. This makes the nipple and areola stand out better.

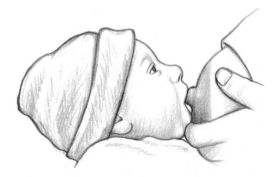

Lower-lip flip.

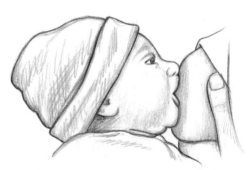

Latch-on.

- Try a recently developed latch-on technique called the asymmetrical latch. Have baby approach the breast chin first from slightly below. Point your nipple upward toward the palate in the back of baby's mouth. Be sure baby's lower jaw covers more of the areola than the upper jaw does. This allows baby's tongue and lower jaw to more effectively massage the areolar tissue below the nipple.
- If baby needs encouragement to open his mouth wide, use the index finger of your hand that is supporting the breast to press down gently on baby's chin as he latches on. (Ask a helper to do this for you at first.) You can keep that index finger on baby's chin throughout the feeding to help him stay on the breast.
- To give baby more support while he is sucking, take the index finger of your hand that is supporting the breast and curve it under baby's chin.
- Get your milk flowing before latching baby onto the breast. When the milk is right there, baby will be more motivated to suck. If you have an abundant milk supply, the strong flow of milk will compensate for baby's weak sucking.
- If multiple attempts at latching on are leading to frustration for you and/or baby, take a break. Your helper can

hold and quiet your baby while you take a few deep breaths and think about something else for a few minutes.

I learned that it does take time. For me it was not innate. It took us three months of trying before he really learned to latch on and nurse.

◆

He was so slow to learn suck-swallow-breathe coordination. Expect to have many training sessions before your baby latches on efficiently.

Nipple shields. Lactation specialists have found that babies who are having difficulty latching onto their mother's bare breast may be able to latch on better if she uses a nipple shield, a thin, flexible silicone nipple that fits over her own nipple. When baby latches onto a bare breast, he must pull the nipple far back into his mouth, to the place where the hard and soft palate meet. This stimulates effective sucking and compression of the milk ducts. It can be difficult for a preemie to accomplish this and to keep the nipple elongated and far back in his mouth throughout the feeding. A nipple shield does some of this work for baby.

If your baby is having trouble latching onto the breast or staying on the breast, consider using a nipple shield. Your lactation consultant or the nursery nurses can help you obtain a silicone shield and determine the size that will work best in your baby's mouth. (How the shield fits in baby's mouth is more important than how it fits your breast.)

To put the shield on your breast, flip the rim up and fit the nipple over your nipple. Then smooth the rim over your

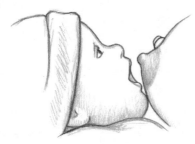

Asymmetrical latch-on.

areola. Dampening the inside of the shield with water or expressed milk will help keep it in place.

When baby latches onto the shield, his tongue and jaws will draw your nipple into his mouth along with the shield nipple. Baby's jaws will compress your breast through the nipple shield, and your milk will flow into baby's mouth through the holes in the shield. You must still pay careful attention to how baby latches on, even with a shield in place.

Because the breast gets less stimulation through the nipple shield, watch your milk supply closely and pay careful attention to how much milk baby is getting at the breast. (As the mother of a preemie, you'll be doing this anyway.) You may need to pump after feedings at first to ensure that your breasts continue to produce enough milk.

You and your baby may end up using the shield for only a few days or for many weeks, depending on your baby's age, anatomy, and development, along with the shape and size of your nipples. Sometimes a preemie's mouth simply has to grow bigger before he can handle Mom's bare breast. If using a nipple shield means your baby can feed at the breast rather than getting supplements from another source, then go ahead and use the shield until baby outgrows the need.

Supplementary feedings. Learning bottlefeeding and breastfeeding at the same time may be confusing for your preemie. The latch-on and sucking techniques used to get milk from an artificial nipple do not work at the breast and the resulting nipple confusion can be very frustrating for both mother and baby. Talk to your baby's caregivers about how baby will be fed when you are not there to breastfeed. Let them know that breastfeeding is important to you and that you want to avoid nipple confusion. Request that your baby continue to receive tube feedings during the time that he is learning to nurse at the breast.

Also, plan to be at the hospital as much as possible when baby is learning to breastfeed, so that you can give baby lots of opportunity to practice. Let the nurses know when you plan to be there so that they avoid filling baby's tummy right before your arrival.

Continuing with tube feedings is only one way to avoid bottle nipples in the neonatal nursery. Other ways of feeding supplements include cup feeding, syringe or eyedropper feeding, finger feeding, or even a spoon.

- *Finger feeding.* This method uses a tube and nursing supplementer to deliver milk to baby as he sucks on an adult finger. The tubing is taped to the caregiver's finger and the finger is inserted into baby's mouth. If the baby is sucking well, milk is drawn through the tube and into his mouth. If baby needs encouragement, the caregiver can squirt a few drops of milk into baby's mouth to stimulate or reward his attempts to suck.
- *Syringe feeding.* The tip of the feeding syringe is inserted between the corner of baby's mouth and the breast. When baby sucks, a few "reward drops" can be squirted into her mouth. Baby can also syringe-feed while sucking on a finger.
- *Cup feeding.* Studies have found that this low-tech approach to giving supplements

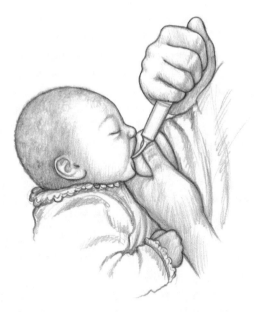

and sucks, she gets the supplement along with the milk from the breast. Meanwhile, baby's sucking helps build the mother's milk supply. As the amount of milk that baby takes from her mother increases, the amount of supplement she drinks at each feeding decreases.

Supplementers are helpful for mothers whose own milk supply is low and for babies who cannot suck strongly enough to get much milk from the breast. The quicker flow of milk from the supplementer will encourage baby to keep nursing. A nursing supplementer is a good way to give your baby supplements after the two of you return home. With the nursing supplementer, baby gets the supplement at the same time she is getting milk from the breast. This eliminates the time and effort it takes to give baby additional milk after feedings at the breast.

does not overstress premature babies and that it works in preemies as young as 30 weeks old. Milk is placed in a small cup, and the caregiver holds baby upright on her lap. The cup is raised to baby's lips so that he can lap or sip the milk. Be careful not to pour the milk into his mouth, which could cause him to choke and wheeze. Cup feeding is used in many countries around the world but is less familiar in American hospitals. One disadvantage of cup feeding is that some of the milk spills or drips down baby's chin and is wasted.

- *Nursing supplementers.* Nursing supplementers are used to give extra milk to baby while she nurses at the breast. The extra milk is poured into a container that hangs from a cord around the mother's neck. Narrow tubing runs from the container to the mother's areola, where it is held in place with tape. (It is possible to use the tubing in conjunction with a nipple shield.) When baby latches on

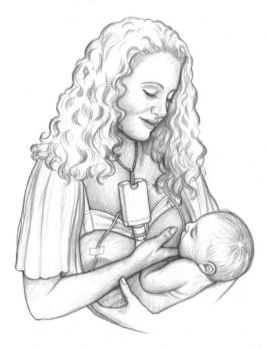

IS BABY GETTING ENOUGH MILK?

As baby's latch-on skills grow, you can begin to focus on how much milk baby is getting while feeding at your breast.

How to Tell

You will know that your baby is getting milk when you hear him swallowing during feedings, after every one or two nutritive sucks. You may notice milk leaking from his mouth after your milk-ejection reflex sends a greater amount of milk down to the nipple, and your breasts will feel softer after feedings. These signs tell you that baby is getting milk, but they don't tell you how much. And sometimes knowing how much is important.

Precise calculations of how much milk baby takes during a breastfeeding can be made using a technique called test weighing. Baby is weighed before the feeding on a sensitive electronic scale and the weight is recorded. Baby is weighed again after the feeding, wearing the same clothes and the same diaper. The number of grams baby gained during the feeding equals the number of milliliters of milk taken in.

Test weighing may confirm your own hunches about how well baby is or is not nursing, or perhaps the results will surprise you. "Test" is an unfortunate choice of words here: there is no grade, no passing or failing. Test weighing simply yields information that you and your baby's caregivers can use to teach your baby to breastfeed better or to decide how much supplement he needs so that he will continue to grow well as he makes the transition to full breastfeeding. (See page 110 for more about supplementary feedings.)

Getting More Milk into Your Baby

One way to enable your baby to nurse longer and take more milk is through a technique called breast compression. When your baby stops sucking, breast compression gets the milk flowing again. Milk in baby's mouth stimulates more sucking.

Here's what to do: When baby's sucking slows down during a feeding, cup your breast between your thumb and fingers. Then hold your breast as close to your chest wall as possible and press your thumb and fingers together — firmly, but not so hard that it hurts. Maintain the pressure while baby resumes active sucking. When his sucking slows or stops, release the pressure. If baby does not resume sucking, rotate the hand and compress a different area of the breast. Baby must be awake and alert when you use this technique. You should not force milk into the mouth of a drowsy or sleeping preemie.

Pumping after feedings will help you maintain a good milk supply (or rebuild one that has dwindled) during the time your baby is learning to breastfeed. When you have an ample milk supply, your milk-ejection reflex can better push more milk down to baby. Then baby gets more milk with less work.

Besides being sure baby gets a large enough volume of milk, it's important to give your baby enough calories. By stimulating your milk-ejection reflex, you can often increase the delivery of grow milk to your baby. Since preemies need extra calories for catch-up growth, here are some tricks of the trade that will enable you to give your baby milk that is higher in fat content and therefore higher in calories.

Finish the breast. Since the calorie content of the milk goes up as the feeding goes on, babies get more high-fat milk the longer and more effectively they nurse. Encourage your baby to keep nursing and "finish" one breast before ending the feeding or switching sides.

Feed often. Studies show that the fat content of milk decreases as the time between feedings increases. If you offer the breast again a half hour or so after baby finishes nursing, she will get another dose of high-fat milk.

Relax your milk in. Breastfeeding, especially breastfeeding a preemie, is a "confidence game." Relaxing your mind and body will help you make more milk. Stress, on the other hand, can inhibit your MER. In one study, mothers of preemies were able to increase their milk delivery by more than 60 percent after listening to a twenty-minute tape on relaxation and visual imagery.

Think baby — think milk. The MER is a conditioned response. That's why you may leak when you just look at or think about your baby (or your pump). While you are breastfeeding, imagine yourself flowing with milk and your baby growing because of your milk.

Massage your MER. Use the breast massage routine described in the pumping section before you feed your baby. (See Perking Up Your Milk Supply, page 99.)

Feed last milk first. You can increase the fat content of the pumped milk that is given to your baby by switching to a new collection bottle midway through your pumping session. The second bottle will contain hindmilk, milk with a higher concentration of fat, which packs more calories into less volume. You or baby's caregivers can feed this "grow milk" when supplementing breastfeeds. Pumping immediately after breastfeeding your baby is another way to obtain milk with a higher fat concentration.

Separate the cream. When you refrigerate your expressed milk, the cream rises to the top. Skim this off and give this to your baby first. Discuss with your doctor, nurse, or lactation consultant the possibility of doing a "creamatocrit." In this procedure, the high-fat hindmilk separates, so that you see what percentage of your milk contains high-fat content. Not only can you then give baby the skimmed-off cream, but this gives you and the staff an idea of the fat content of your milk and the effectiveness of the above ways to increase it. Remember, your baby needs your "whole milk," not just the cream. Although hindmilk is higher in fat, and therefore calories, your baby also needs the nutrients that are more plentiful in the milk released earlier in the feeding. Just seeing that layer of rich grow milk may give you a boost as your realize that your milk truly is the best medicine.

Eat the right fats to make the right fats. The fats you eat can influence the fats in the milk you make. The best fats for growing brains are LC-PUFAs, especially DHA (discussed on page 85). The best dietary sources of LC-PUFAs are seafood, such as wild salmon. Another rich source is "omega eggs," eggs from free-range chickens whose feed is high in omega-3s, one of two essential fatty acids (EFAs), so called because they are essential for life and health. EFAs form the building blocks of vital cell membranes and are used to manufacture important substances, such as hormones. You can also get omega-3 LC-PUFAs in flaxseed oil (1 tablespoon a day of the oil or two tablespoons a day of ground flaxseeds mixed in a fruit-and-yogurt smoothie). However, the complex biochemical process that turns omega-3s from plant sources into DHA may not always operate at peak efficiency in your body. For this reason, it's best to get your omega 3s directly from a marine source. If you don't like seafood, purchase a supplement called Neuromins, which contains a purified form of DHA made from marine plants. (For more information about the safest and richest sources of omega-3 fats for the breastfeeding mother, see www.askdrsears.com/preemies.)

BREASTFEEDING YOUR PREEMIE AT HOME

While you're happy to be taking your preemie home at last, you may be a bit apprehensive about feeding your baby without your helpers around. In the first days of being on their own, most mothers (even mothers of full-term babies) worry about whether their baby is getting enough milk. As you see your baby grow and thrive, this anxiety will go away. In the meantime, here's how to make the transition from hospital to home easier on your baby and yourself.

Consult your team. Before you leave the hospital, be sure you get all your questions about home feedings answered. The

> ### RECOMMENDED BREASTFEEDING VIDEO
>
> *A Preemie Needs His Mother — First Steps to Breastfeeding Your Premature Baby,* produced by Jane Murton, M.D., is a two-part video series that shows parents the value of breastfeeding a preemie. It includes instructions on how to pump and store breast milk, as well as how to teach baby to breastfeed and how to transition from gavage feeding. It is available from Stanford Breastfeeding Medicine Program, 750 Welch Road, Suite 315, Palo Alto, CA 94304, or through La Leche League International.

questions you have will depend upon whether your baby is getting all of her milk at the breast or some of it another way (e.g., you are supplementing with your pumped milk or "combo feeding" with breast milk and formula). Write down questions as you think of them in the days before baby is ready to leave the hospital. Take advantage of all your consultants while they are nearby.

Get professional help. If you and baby need a hands-on refresher course in proper latch-on and breastfeeding, we recommend you hire a certified lactation consultant (LC) to come over for a home visit (see Resources, page 235). Not only can she help you get baby latched on properly, but she can also answer questions about pumping and help you set up your breastfeeding "nest" at home so that you are comfortable in your own environment.

If your baby was not yet breastfeeding well when you left the hospital, then you really need to invest in the help of a lactation consultant who knows preemies well if you want to breastfeed in the months to come. You will probably need several visits with the lactation consultant. Your health insurance may cover the cost of LC visits if your doctor writes a letter stating that they are medically necessary. Your insurance company may be more willing to pay for follow-up visits with the hospital's lactation consultants than for services from an LC in private practice. If you cannot afford a private lactation consultant and your insurance doesn't cover it, some hospitals have a breastfeeding clinic that you can attend for a fraction of the cost. When considering the cost of services from a lactation consultant, remember that breastfeeding can eventually save you money. Getting the help you need to make breastfeeding work for your baby will be worth it in the long run.

Create a peaceful nest. Wouldn't it be nice if you could arrive home with your baby, walk into a spotless house, sit down in your rocking chair in your pastel-painted nursery with soft sunlight filtering through the window, and magically nurse your little baby to sleep? While such a perfect picture may not be possible, we suggest you do set up a comfortable spot in your home where you can relax and focus on breastfeeding. This will include a favorite chair, a footstool, lots of pillows, a table for drinks and snacks, music, and anything else you might need.

Welcome a home nurse visit. Many hospitals offer a home visit by a nurse a day or two after you leave the NICU. She can answer any questions you have and reassure you that baby is doing fine.

Nurse your preemie frequently. Preemies have tiny tummies that hold only small meals. If you follow your baby's cues and offer the breast when he squirms, roots, or seems hungry, you will probably find that you are nursing at least every two hours during the day. Studies have shown that the fat content of a mother's milk increases as the time between feedings decreases. This means that frequent feedings are the best strategy for getting the highest-calorie milk into baby.

If baby takes long daytime naps, you may need to wake him for some feedings. If he's been asleep for two to three hours, start watching for signs of restlessness, an indication that he is moving from one sleep stage to another and could be awakened easily. Don't let your preemie go more than two or three hours during the day or four or five hours during the night without a feeding.

Sling feed. Between regular feedings, wear your baby in a sling as you walk around the house or do chores. Being inches away from his favorite food may entice him to eat more. You can feed your baby right in the sling. Some preemies suck better while mother is moving gently.

Respect your baby's signals. You need to find a balance between frequent feeding and baby's need for sleep and rest. During the first weeks at home, you will spend much of your time feeding your baby, giving supplements, and pumping to keep up your milk supply. Plan on keeping baby close to you during the day — in the sling or in your arms. While frequent feeding is important, baby also needs time to experience the peacefulness of just being near you, without having to deal with the challenges of feeding.

Reward yourself for all the effort you are putting into breastfeeding by savoring the wonderful feeling of holding your baby in your arms. Gaze into his eyes when he's awake, caress his soft head with your cheek when he's asleep. This is your baby, and despite a difficult beginning, the two of you now share the unique bond of breastfeeding.

FEEDING QUESTIONS YOU MAY HAVE

How much milk should baby get?

Many preemies do not give consistent cues "demanding" to breastfeed, so it is helpful to know how much milk your baby needs to keep growing at a good pace. We know that babies need about 2½ to 3 ounces of milk for each pound of body weight per day, but when baby is exclusively or mostly breastfeeding, how can you make sure baby is getting enough? The single most accurate way to know a baby is getting enough nutrition is to monitor the weight gain. But it is impossible to take baby to the doctor's office every few days for a weight check. You may be able to rent an electronic scale for several weeks for use at home, and seeing baby pile on the ounces will reassure you. Renting a scale also allows you to do "test weighs" on baby (see page 112).

A research study of sixty mothers of preemies showed that those who did test weighs at home had significantly less anxiety about their babies' milk intake than those who did not. Doing test weighs with each feeding for a whole day can give you a good idea of baby's intake.

However, it is almost impossible to measure the exact number of ounces that an exclusively breastfed infant is taking in, even with test weighing. If your baby is feeding well at the breast and showing proof of this through adequate weight gain, then supplementation may no longer be necessary. If, on the other hand, baby is nursing well but not gaining weight as he should, it is likely that he isn't getting enough milk with each feed. There are two ways to approach this situation, whether baby is in the NICU or at home.

Top baby off. Allow baby to feed at the breast on cue approximately every two hours. After each nursing, offer baby a small amount of pumped breast milk or formula from a bottle, syringe, cup, or feeding tube (see Supplementary Feedings, page 110). If baby did not quite get enough from the breast, he may eagerly take in a bit more. If, on the other hand, baby did get a full tummy from the breast, he may reject any supplement that you offer. Doing this after each feeding will help make sure baby gets what he needs.

There are some drawbacks to this system. It takes more time and effort to prepare a supplement after each feeding. While in the NICU, the nurses will help with this, but once you go home, you may find this task overwhelming. In addition, filling baby up or overfeeding him may make him so full that he won't want to

NAP NURSING

Your preemie is waking frequently during the night to nurse. You're exhausted and you're worried that baby may not be getting enough milk. Here's a trick we call nap nursing that can ease both of these concerns. At least two times a day, lie down to breastfeed your baby. Chances are, you'll both catch a nap. And since the levels of milk-producing hormones go up when you sleep, you're likely to deliver more milk to your baby as well. Babies enjoy the peace and quiet of nap nursing and are likely to breastfeed more eagerly and longer. They may doze for a while and then wake up for another helping of the high-fat "grow milk" that remains in mother's breasts when the intervals between feedings are short. The side-lying position, similar to night nursing, is usually best for nap nursing. Cradle your baby in your arm while you both lie on your side facing each other. Use a pillow behind your lower back to help you relax your whole body. Play relaxing music. Take the phone off the hook.

We have used this technique for many years in our pediatric practice to boost the growth of infants, especially preemies, and help tired mothers take a break during the day. If baby gets more milk during daylight hours, he may be less likely to wake up so often at night.

As you get into a nap nursing routine, you'll notice that baby eagerly anticipates these special feedings. While it's tempting to get up and "get something done" once baby is asleep, resist the urge. When you are nap-nursing, you are doing one of the most important jobs in the world: growing a human being.

nurse again for several hours. This will decrease his overall time at the breast, which can have an adverse effect on your overall milk supply. There may be a better option. Read on.

Catch-up feeds. Allow baby to feed on cue at the breast throughout an extended period of time (eight to twelve hours) without any supplementation. At the end of each time period, offer baby some catch-up supplemental feedings of either pumped breast milk or formula. While baby is still in the NICU, you can allow her to rest from all that vigorous breast-feeding and have the nurse give her some gavage feeds through a feeding tube.

Once you are home, use whatever alternative feeding system works best for you and your baby.

The number of ounces needed to "catch up" is not always clear. It all comes down to weight gain. Give as much supplement as needed to achieve the desired weight gain day by day. A rented electronic scale is invaluable during this time. Doing test weighs with every feeding for an eight- to twelve-hour period is one way to approximate how many ounces or milliliters baby took in. Then you will know approximately how much catch-up supplementation baby may need for that period. For example, your 3-pound baby needs about 8 or 9 ounces per day, or 3 ounces every eight hours. Baby feeds three times in an eight-hour period. Test weighs with each feeding show baby gains 1 ounce, ½ ounce, and 1 ounce. This totals 2½ ounces for that eight-hour period. You would then supplement with ½ ounce to achieve the 3-ounce goal.

With this method, babies get supplements only two or three times a day rather than after every feeding. It's easier for babies to make the transition to cue feeding and to regulating their own intake when Mom or Dad is not filling them up with supplement after every feeding. And you will spend less time preparing and giving supplemental feedings. As baby's breastfeeding skills improve and weight gain is sufficient, you can slowly cut back on how much supplement you offer.

How often should I breastfeed my baby?

While we usually recommend feeding on cue for a full-term baby, your preemie may still be too sleepy and too young to ask for a feeding every two to three hours. (See below for an explanation of "feeding on cue.") If you waited for your preemie to ask to be fed, she might go six hours before her hunger bothered her enough to make her needs known. That's why we suggest you start with a combination of feeding on cue and following a flexible schedule similar to what was working well for baby in the NICU. If your baby shows signs of hunger one or one and a half hours after the last feeding, by all means go ahead and feed her. If more than three hours go by and baby doesn't ask to feed, then you initiate the feeding. (It's okay to go three to four hours between feedings at night if baby will allow it.) Most pree-

---

> ## GUIDELINES FOR WEIGHT GAIN
>
> As a general guide, an optimal weight gain for a preemie at home is approximately 1 ounce a day. Each day, preemies should gain about ¼ ounce for every pound they weigh (or 15 grams for every kilogram). Therefore, a 2-pound preemie (1 kilogram) in the NICU is expected to gain about ½ ounce (or 15 grams) each day. A 4-pound baby (2 kilograms) who is ready to go home should be gaining about 1 ounce (30 grams) each day. Babies may gain less one day and more the next, but there should be adequate weight gain over a week's time.

---

mies welcome the more frequent feedings they get at home, when Mom-nurse doesn't have to follow a hospital routine. Try not to let your baby go longer between feedings than she did in the NICU. If the NICU was feeding your baby every two or three hours, use this as the maximum time between feedings, with some feedings occurring sooner if baby asks. Keep in mind that *there's no such thing as breastfeeding your baby too often*. Keeping a breastfed preemie on a strict three- or four-hour schedule puts baby at risk for failure to thrive, a serious condition in which baby does not grow physically, emotionally, and developmentally.

What does "feeding on cue" mean?

Pediatricians used to use the term "feeding on demand" to describe when to breastfeed baby, but we feel this isn't the best way to explain what goes on between mother and baby. "Feeding on demand" implies that you must wait until your baby demands to be fed by fussing or crying. Crying is a very late sign of hunger — and a waste of energy. By the time a baby cries to be fed, he has probably already been hungry for a while. We encourage you instead to learn your baby's early hunger cues. These may include rooting (turning the head back and forth and looking for something to suck on), sucking on the fingers or hand, squirming, kicking the hands and feet, following you with her eyes, and vocalization. Of course, these activities won't *always* mean your baby is hungry, and that's where intuitive parenting comes in. Over time, you will learn which cues mean "feed me, please," and which ones mean something else. But in these early stages, don't hesitate to offer baby the breast.

How can I tell if my baby is getting enough breast milk?

In the NICU, your baby was weighed every day. As long as he was gaining enough weight, the medical staff were confident that your baby was getting enough calories. The nurses also kept track of how much breast milk or formula baby received by bottlefeeding or tube-feeding. You and the nurses may even have used test weighing (weighing baby before and after breastfeeding) to determine how much milk baby took from the breast.

But now you are on your own. Unless you are using a scale to do test weighs at home, you have no way to tell how much milk baby is getting. Here are some signs you can watch for that will reassure you baby is feeding well:

Number of wet diapers. As a general guide, baby should have six to eight wet diapers a day. Before you leave the NICU, make yourself familiar with how often baby urinates.

Stooling pattern. If baby's stool pattern is similar to what it was while he was growing well in the NICU, this is a good sign. Over the next few months, baby's stools may become less frequent as his intestines become more efficient at digesting breast milk. If baby's stooling slows down considerably in the first week or two after you come home, check baby's weight gain (see next page).

Stool color. Yellow, seedy stools (resembling gourmet mustard) are typical of breastfed babies. If baby produced these in the NICU but most of her stools are becoming more liquid, green, or mucusy, this may mean baby's intake has decreased.

That contented look. A baby who has just filled his tummy with breast milk will often have a satisfied, almost drunk look. On the other hand, a baby who has not gotten enough may still act hungry and fuss and keep wanting to nurse. However, after-feeding behaviors are the least reliable signs of whether or not baby is getting enough milk. Babies with reflux fuss after feeding, yet they may be getting sufficient milk. Some preemies with weak sucking patterns may not get enough milk but may fall asleep after feeding because they are tired.

Weight gain. This is the most accurate way for you to know baby is getting enough milk. You have three choices. You can just go by how you think baby feels and looks; you can take baby to the pediatrician for weight checks once or twice a week; or you can rent an electronic infant scale from the hospital, a lactation consultant, or a health equipment company. Renting a scale may save you from a lot of driving around town, but be careful that "watching the numbers" doesn't keep you from enjoying your baby. You may find that monitoring baby's weight closely at home, doing test weighs before and after feedings, actually helps you worry less. Decide which method of weight watching fits you best. Don't worry if baby doesn't seem to gain weight over one or two days. It's the weight gain over several days that matters. Also, be aware that all scales measure differently. Baby's first weight at home or at the pediatrician's office may measure lower than the NICU discharge weight. Use the first weight on a given scale as a starting point and monitor baby's weight gain with the same scale from this point on.

When can I begin exclusive breastfeeding?

This is a long-term goal that a lactation consultant and your doctor can help you achieve. If you stop supplemental feedings too soon, you can put your baby at risk of inadequate weight gain. The age at which babies achieve exclusive breastfeeding depends on many factors. Expert help and your own instincts as parents can help you reach your goal.

Learning more. Pumping and breastfeeding your baby in the neonatal nursery is only the beginning of the adventure. For more information on breastfeeding babies as they grow and change, read our *Breastfeeding Book* (see Resources, page 235).

Bottlefeeding Your Preemie

FEEDING YOUR BABY is about more than just milk.* Bottlefeeding, like breastfeeding, is a time for social interaction. Regardless of what kind of milk your infant gets or where it comes from, be sure your baby knows the milk is coming from *you*. Filling their tummies makes babies feel good, and you want your baby to associate these good feelings with human contact, in much the same way as you enjoy celebrating friendships with a good meal.

In this chapter you will learn about both the art and the science of bottlefeeding, which formula to choose, and how to deliver it to baby so that feeding is a pleasant experience for both of you. Whether you are bottlefeeding exclusively or combining bottlefeeding with breastfeeding, you'll soon learn that there's more involved than just inserting the nipple into baby's mouth. Here are common

questions asked by parents of bottlefeeding preemies.

FIRST FEEDINGS

When can my baby begin to take a bottle?

The day you get the green light to go ahead and begin bottlefeeding your preemie is an exciting one. Finally you can sit quietly in a rocking chair with baby cradled in your arms and gaze at your baby while she feels safe, warm, and well fed. Yet, if you had visions of baby eagerly sucking away at the bottle and downing several ounces quickly, think again. It will take time for your little one to be able to really "chow down." Most preemies can begin bottlefeeding between 32 and 34 weeks' gestation, the age at which most preemies begin to coordinate sucking, swallowing, and breathing. Your baby's medical situation and level of maturity will dictate when he is ready to make the transition from gavage feeding to nipple feeding. Because babies tire easily during bottlefeeding, it's important to wait until baby

---

* In this section we are using the term "milk" to mean both pumped breast milk and commercial infant formula. The bottlefeeding advice in this chapter will be helpful for both mothers who "combo feed" (breast and bottle) and mothers who exclusively formula-feed their babies.

no longer needs mechanical assistance with breathing and is breathing comfortably on her own. In NICU speak, once baby is "tolerating gavage feedings well," "off the vent," and "out of the oxy-hood," baby can begin "nippling." Once you hear the nurses mention nipple feeding, get ready.

SPECIAL PRECAUTIONS

What special precautions do I need to take in bottlefeeding my preemie?

Sucking, swallowing, and breathing — what a baby needs to do to feed — are instinctive, but it is hard work for baby to learn to coordinate these three actions. The goal is for baby to be able to get the most milk with the least amount of work. The more energy baby can conserve while feeding, the more energy he has to grow. Here's how you can help baby become an expert at sucking and swallowing and breathing all at the same time:

Watch baby suck. Babies begin to suck at around 28 weeks. Their first sucking is very gentle, but the intensity gradually increases as baby grows. To prepare baby to get her food by sucking, let her practice sucking on your well-scrubbed finger or on a pacifier. Your baby's nurses may encourage her to suck during nasogastric tube feedings so that she will begin to associate sucking with filling her tummy. Sucking stimulates the production of saliva, so it also encourages baby to practice swallowing.

If you are planning to combine breastfeeding and bottlefeeding, encourage your baby to suck on your nipples before introducing her to bottle nipples. Not only

---

THE FEEDING SEQUENCE

Expect feeding methods to change as baby's sucking, swallowing, and digestive mechanisms mature:

- *28 weeks and younger:* intravenous fluids plus TPN (total parenteral nutrition), which means all of baby's nutrients are supplied intravenously; start trophic feeds (tiny drip-milk feeds that help baby's stomach and intestines mature)
- *28 to 34 weeks:* intravenous fluids, TPN, plus gavage feedings
- *32 to 37 weeks:* gavage feedings plus feeding by breast, bottle, nursing supplementer, cup, or syringe
- *after 37 weeks:* usually breast or bottle only

Preemies' stage of development determines how they are fed. Babies do not manufacture the enzymes needed to digest milk until around 28 to 30 weeks' gestation. This is why very young preemies are limited to intravenous nutrition, which passes the stomach entirely. Once the stomach is ready for milk, tube feedings bypass the mouth, until the suck-swallow-breathe sequence begins to click in between 32 and 34 weeks of age. Decisions about how your baby is fed will also take into account his medical situation.

---

does this promote bonding, but it may also be easier on baby. Research has shown that babies tire less when sucking during breastfeeding than they do during bottlefeeding. Babies can usually start sucking from mother's breast about two weeks before they are ready to suck milk from a bottle. Baby may naturally try to suck at your breast during kangaroo care. We have cared for adopting mothers who eagerly used their breasts as pacifiers for their preemies, even before baby was ready to take the bottle nipple. Sucking on your finger, empty breast, or a pacifier is called nonnutritive sucking. (For information on the benefits of nonnutritive sucking, see page 105.)

Watch baby swallow. Your baby has been swallowing his saliva since birth, so certainly he knows how to swallow, but he is accustomed to swallowing only a few drops of saliva at a time. This is why bottlefeedings begin with a few drops rather than a few ounces. One concern related to swallowing is the development of baby's gag reflex, which is what keeps food or liquid out of the lungs when he makes the mistake of breathing and swallowing at the same time. Babies usually don't develop a mature gag reflex until around 34 or 35 weeks' gestation. If your baby gets too much formula too fast and the gag reflex does not protest the excess, it's possible for formula to enter baby's lungs (through aspiration) and irritate them. (This is less of a concern with breastfeeding. Mother's milk usually does not flow very fast during early feedings, especially if she has pumped before putting baby to the breast, and since breast milk is a natural human substance, it does not irritate the lining of the breathing passages if a few drops are aspirated into the lungs. It's necessary to be more cautious when formula-feeding a preemie than when breastfeeding.) Since very premature infants typically don't know how

to swallow very well, expect to see milk dribble out of baby's mouth during these first feedings. If pumped breast milk is in the bottle, you may cringe at seeing the milk go to waste. Yet, rest assured: much more ends up going into baby's stomach than dribbles out. Baby will soon learn to manage more milk in the mouth during each feeding. Take dribbling as a sign that you and baby need to slow down.

Watch baby breathe. Baby needs to learn the secret of breathing between swallows and swallowing between breaths. Because preemies usually breathe so fast, neonatologists prefer to wait until baby's respiratory rate is below sixty breaths per minute before starting bottlefeedings. If baby is puffing along at a respiratory rate faster than this, there is not much time between breaths for baby to swallow. Typically, baby will take a few sucks to fill his mouth, swallow, and then take several quick breaths. Baby will eventually learn to suck *and* breathe at the same time, and then hold his breath briefly to swallow. With beginning bottlefeeding, expect dribbles, sputters, chokes, and gags. These preemie feeding quirks even occur when veteran NICU nurses give bottlefeedings. With practice, baby will learn to properly coordinate breathing and swallowing.

Dr. Bill advises: Feeding a preemie is an exercise in baby-reading. Bottlefeeding term babies is relatively easy, and you don't have to pay that much attention to the suck-swallowbreathe coordination. Term babies just do it. Preemies must learn how, and parents must watch. While certainly it's more challenging to feed a preemie, you could actually consider it a perk. The increased focused attention you give your baby during feeding is simply another opportunity for you to study your baby. You'll learn when to slow down, when to take a break, and when to go with the good feeding rhythm baby has established. Fast-forward this tape a couple years: One day you'll be at a birthday party with your toddler and you'll know when she's had enough fun and it's time to think about going home, gracefully, before the public meltdown. That knowledge of your child began in a rocking chair in the NICU.

SPECIAL TECHNIQUES

Are there special techniques and equipment I need to bottlefeed my preemie?

Because your baby has a smaller mouth, a smaller tummy, and weaker oral muscles, think "small" and "slow" when it comes to bottlefeeding him. Plenty of patience helps, too. Here are some tips from NICU nurses and parents of preemies:

Use preemie bottles and nipples. You may notice that the bottles and nipples used in the NICU are about half the size of the ones you've seen before. That's because your baby may be half the size of the other babies. Preemie nipples tend to be shorter and softer and have a slower flow rate. When you hold the full bottle upside down, milk should drip from the nipple at a rate of around one drop per second. Your baby's nurse will choose and change the bottle and the nipples according to your baby's degree of prematurity

and progress in feeding. By discharge day, your baby will probably be using standard 4-ounce bottles with medium-flow nipples.

Preemie bottles are usually calibrated in cubic centimeters (cc's) or in milliliters (ml's). Five cc or 5 ml equal 1 teaspoon, and 30 ml equal 1 ounce. While milk volume is usually measured in ounces in term babies, it's usually measured in cc's or ml's in preemies, something you will grow accustomed to in the NICU.

To minimize the amount of air baby swallows during feedings, try nursers that hold the milk in a disposable bag that collapses during feeding. Or try angled bottles, which allow the air to rise to the top of the bottle while the entire bottom stays covered with milk. Swallowing air is hard on preemies, since a gas-filled tummy can press upward on the diaphragm and further compromise breathing.

Teach baby how to suck better. While sucking is instinctual, baby's nurse will show you some tricks of the trade to get baby to suck and swallow more efficiently. If your baby sleeps more than sucks, the nurse will show you how to stimulate or tickle his cheeks or lips to remind baby to keep feeding. Veteran NICU nurses use the "cheek squeeze" to help babies feed more efficiently. Gently squeeze baby's cheeks between your thumb and forefinger to stimulate baby to suck. Squeezing the cheeks forward purses the lips open wider and stimulates sucking. To help baby "milk" the bottle nipple, use a finger to gently press upward just behind baby's chin. The combination of the cheek squeeze and chin support compresses the nipple between baby's tongue and palate. Instead of the traditional cradle hold during bottlefeeding, hold baby upright on your lap.

If you are combo feeding (both breast and bottle), a lactation consultant may have some other tricks to show you about bottlefeeding. She can show you how to position baby's mouth and lips around the bottle nipple in a manner similar to proper latch-on at the breast. This may help baby avoid nipple confusion.

Slow the feeds, but not too much. The goal when feeding a preemie is for baby to take in the most milk while using the least energy. While you need to feed your baby slowly enough to prevent gagging and choking, you don't want him to waste energy fighting for his food or taking forever to finish a feed. For beginning bottle-feeders, twenty- to thirty-minute feedings are the goal. If baby takes to bottlefeeding eagerly and sucks efficiently, then you can adjust the time and frequency of the feeding accordingly. During the first week or so of bottlefeeding, expect your preemie to continue with gavage feeding as well. Giving some feedings by gavage ensures that baby gets enough to eat during the transition to nipple feeding and doesn't expend too much energy on eating. At first baby will be given a couple bottle-feedings a day and the rest of the feedings will be given through a tube. Later she will be bottlefed at each feeding and "topped off" several times a day with additional milk by gavage in order to be sure she is getting enough to eat that day. (See Gavage Feeding, next page.)

Set baby up to feed. One way to help babies or small children feel less anxious about transitioning into a different activity is to use a "setting event." An enjoyable stimulus — the setting event — sets baby up for a predictable effect. For example, cuddling your toddler in your arms and singing your toddler a familiar lullaby sets him up for drifting off to sleep. To get your baby in an alert mood for bottlefeeding, choose an interaction your baby enjoys — her favorite touch, her favorite song, a few drops of milk on her lips — and offer these right before a feeding. Gentle touching is an especially good way to prepare baby for a feeding, since preemies often learn to associate kangaroo care with sucking. The general ambiance of Mother or Father's body, the voice, touch, and smell remind them of the pleasures of feeding. It's similar to the experience of walking into your favorite restaurant and discovering that you are a lot hungrier than you thought. Experiment until you discover what kind of stimulation best readies your preemie for feeding sessions. Too much touching and talking and your baby will be revved up to the point where he wastes energy and can't concentrate on feeding; too little stimulation and he will fall asleep as he sucks. But just the right amount will keep him awake and interested.

HOW MUCH? HOW OFTEN?

How much milk should my baby take in, and how often should I feed her?

Preemies seem to need more of every kind of care, and more food is no exception. The special needs of preemies make feeding more challenging: they need more

GAVAGE FEEDING

Preemies younger than 34 weeks' gestation do not have the energy and maturity to coordinate sucking, swallowing, and breathing well enough to get all their nourishment directly from the breast or bottle. So, they are fed by gavage (from the French *gaver,* meaning "to gorge with food"). The nurse gently inserts a soft plastic tube through baby's mouth or nose into the stomach and gives baby milk through the tube. For the very premature infant, the first tube feedings may be trophic feedings, very small amounts of breast milk or dilute formula, and eventually baby may tolerate more breast milk or full-strength formula.

Watching the insertion of a feeding tube may be disturbing to parents, but it doesn't bother babies very much, since infants don't develop a gag reflex until around 34 weeks. The tube is left in place during the time that baby's nourishment is exclusively provided by tube feedings. When baby begins to take milk directly from the breast or bottle, the gavage tube may be left in (called a long-term gavage tube) or reinserted after some feedings to provide extra milk that baby doesn't have to work for. Once baby is strong and mature enough to take all of her milk by breast or bottle, tube feedings are no longer necessary.

You can do it! Watch the nurse "gavage" your baby. The nurse will either attach the end of the tube to a container holding a specified amount of milk and let it drip into baby's tummy or use a syringe attached to a pump to slowly push a measured amount of milk through the tube and into baby's stomach. Then the nurse will record how much milk baby took. Ask the nurse to show you how to hold and manipulate the syringe so that after the tube has been inserted, you can do gavage feedings yourself (with the nurse's assistance). Besides reporting to the nurses how much milk you gave baby, you can also record this information in your own diary.

Encourage sucking while feeding. While baby is receiving tube feedings, let her suck on your finger or place a few drops of whatever milk is in the tube on her tongue. Not only does this help her associate sucking with feeding, but the extra sucking stimulates saliva production, which helps digestion in the stomach and intestines. Remember, no matter how your baby is being fed, feedings should always include social interaction in addition to delivery of milk.

calories for catch-up growth, and, because of their immature digestive system, they need to be fed more often. As a general rule, your preemie will need to eat around 25 percent more calories per day relative to his weight than a newborn term baby does. Yet you can't just put more formula in every bottle. Remember our motto for feeding preemies: More for less! Preemies need more milk with less expenditure of energy. Baby's immature intestines cannot handle big loads. The increased amount of milk your baby needs can be given only by increasing the frequency of feedings. Only as baby gets older can you gradually increase the amount.

We nicknamed our baby "More."

There are several reasons why preemies need to be fed more frequently:

1. Immature digestion. Like most of your preemie's other systems, the digestive system is not yet mature enough to work at top efficiency. Feeding baby slowly, frequently, and in smaller amounts allows for more complete digestion. Otherwise, baby's intestines bog down as they fill with partially digested milk. This results in constipation, colicky abdominal pain, and inadequate nutrition for growth.

2. Reflux. Most premature babies have some degree of gastroesophageal reflux (GERD) (see page 195). Smaller amounts fed slowly but more frequently are digested better, with less food left over to be regurgitated.

3. Bloating. Too much food in the stomach can make it harder for baby to breathe (like the way you may feel as you loosen your belt after Thanksgiving dinner). Undigested food turns to gas, which inflates baby's intestines. This makes it harder for baby's diaphragm to move downward with each breath and thus may compromise his breathing.

4. Energy conservation. When too much food flows too fast, your preemie frantically tries to cope and uses a lot of energy in the process. Preemies enjoy being fed s-l-o-w-l-y, with frequent pauses to rest during the feeding.

How many ounces does my baby need at each feeding?

For optimal growth, by discharge day your preemie needs 2½ to 3 ounces of milk per pound of body weight each day. Tiny babies have tiny tummies, about the size of their fist. An ounce or 2 per feeding doesn't sound like much, but if you place 2 ounces of formula in a bottle and compare the space it takes up with the size of your baby's fist, you will notice the mismatch. As a very general rule, by the time baby is ready for discharge, expect baby's doctor to prescribe the "2–3 feeding guide": 2 ounces every two to three hours. Unless advised otherwise by your baby's doctor, you may not have to awaken your baby for feedings during the night. (Remember, babies grow while sleeping because that's when growth hormone is secreted most.) Just feed him when he wakes. Yet, for the first month or so, don't expect him to sleep for more than a three-hour stretch.

A quick and easy way to figure out how many ounces your baby may need by discharge day is to multiply baby's weight in pounds by 2½ or 3. For example, a 4-pound baby will need around 10 to 12 ounces (300 to 350 cc) of milk per day. If your baby is fed every three hours (eight feeds per day), then your baby will need about 1¼ to 1½ ounces, or 35 to 45 cc (ml), per feeding. In the NICU, the metric system rules. You will hear the nurses talk about baby's feedings in terms of "cc's," which means cubic centimeters, or in "ml's," which means milliliters. A cc is the same amount of liquid as an ml; 1 ounce equals 30 cc or ml. Most full-term babies typically take in 2 to 4 ounces at each feeding in the early months. Your preemie, however, may take in only 1 or 2 ounces per feeding, or 30 to 60 cc. Depending on your preemie's gestational age, the first week or so, he may tolerate only ½ ounce per feeding and graduate to 1 to 2 ounces per feeding by discharge day.

Counting calories. You may think your baby is a little young to be counting calories, but the nursing staff and nutritionists in the NICU will actually be paying very close attention to how many calories your baby is getting every day. The goal for most preemies is 120 to 150 calories per kilogram of body weight (55 to 70 calories per pound) each day. This means that when your baby weighs about 2 kilograms (4 pounds, 2 ounces), he will need 250 to 300 calories per day. Breast milk contains 20 calories per ounce. Formula has varying amounts of calories (from 20 to 24 calories per ounce), depending on the

type being used. If a 2-kilogram baby needs 240 calories per day, he needs 12 ounces of milk per day.

CHOOSING A FORMULA

What type of formula should I feed our preemie?

By the time you leave the hospital, you, the medical staff, and your baby will figure out which formula given in what amount and how frequently is best tolerated by your baby. As babies grow and their medical condition changes, they may need a change in formula. Oftentimes, premature babies need special preemie formulas in the early weeks. As the intestines mature, babies can often graduate to standard infant formulas. Here are the options:

Standard formulas.
- Cow's milk–based formula, including Enfamil, Similac, Carnation Good Start, and generic brands.
- Hypoallergenic or elemental formula, including Nutramigen, Pregestimil, Alimentum, and Neocate. The nutritional components of these formulas are already partially broken down into smaller molecules (predigested) so baby can more easily absorb them. They are used only in special situations when baby isn't tolerating cow's milk formula.

Higher-calorie formulas. Moderately and extremely premature babies are usually started on a specialized formula made to meet their special nutritional needs. These formulas contain slightly higher levels of certain nutrients and come in

---

PREEMIE BOTTLEFEEDING TIPS

- Make feeding a high-touch time of social interaction.
- Offer smaller feedings more frequently.
- Keep baby upright (at least 30 degrees above horizontal) and quiet for at least a half hour after feedings.
- Encourage baby to burp during or after a feeding.
- Feed slowly and allow rest stops.
- Use a DHA/ARA-enriched formula if not using breast milk.
- Keep a feeding diary.

various strengths from 20 to 24 calories per ounce.

Unique growth requirements determine which formula your baby should have, and your neonatologist will help you figure out which one is best for your baby. How long your baby will continue to need a special preemie formula is up to her pediatrician. In general, the younger and smaller baby is at birth, the longer she may need a preemie formula. A 28-week preemie may need it for the entire first year.

Higher-calorie formulas for higher-risk babies. Preemie babies with certain medical problems such as chronic lung disease (see page 184) need even more calories than other preemies do, since they use more energy to breathe and pump blood to the body. So why not just feed them more formula to make up the difference? Preemies can handle only a limited volume of milk. Plus, preemies with lung or heart problems may retain too much water in their bodies if they are given too much formula, causing their hearts to work even harder. With more calories packed into each ounce of formula, your baby can get extra nutrition without risking fluid overload.

Choose formulas enriched with "smart fats." New studies indicate that preemies given formulas enriched with essential fatty acids, both the omega-3 docosahexanoeic acid (DHA) and omega-6 arachidonic acid (ARA), show improved visual acuity and higher scores on developmental tests later in childhood than infants fed formulas not enriched with these fats. This makes sense since omega-3 fats are a prime structural component of the brain and the retina of the eye.

Formula with added DHA and ARA has been available for several years in Europe. Beginning in February of 2002, manufacturers began to market infant formula enriched with these brain-building fats in the United States. However, not all commercial infant formulas contain these essential fats. Research suggests that getting these fats from dietary sources is necessary and not optional for optimal preemie development. New insights into infant nutrition suggest that preemies, and perhaps term infants as well, do not yet have the metabolic ability to transform other fats in their diet into these important substances. Thus, they need to get ready-made smart fats from infant formula. Not surprisingly, these smart fats are found in human milk. They must be there for a reason, since nature makes very few nutritional mistakes. When you select a formula for your baby, choose one that contains these important omega-3 fatty acids, especially if your baby is exclusively formula-fed and not getting these substances from your milk.

FORMULA ALLERGIES

How do I know if a particular formula isn't agreeing with my baby?

Some babies go through many formula changes before mother and doctor discover which one is most intestines friendly. The good news is that as baby's intestines mature, her tummy won't be so picky about the formula it gets. Your baby can't tell you when her tiny tummy is upset, but your observations of how she acts can give you the information you and the doctor require to decide whether she needs a change of formula. Here are some "formula intolerant" signs to watch for:

Spitting up. The stomach and intestines instinctively reject what they don't like. While a bit of spitting up is normal, especially in preemies, spitting up at every feeding with enough force to make the formula go splat all over Mom or Dad could indicate that baby is allergic to the formula. However, spitting up usually has more to do with the feeding technique than the type of formula, especially if baby has reflux. When baby swallows lots of air during a feeding, air bubbles trapped in the stomach can force milk right back up baby's esophagus and out of his mouth. (For tips on feeding a baby with reflux, see page 196.) If your baby spits up large amounts frequently, fiddle with the feeding technique first before changing the type of formula. Feed baby smaller amounts more frequently. If the spitting up subsides, you don't need to try a different formula.

Bloating. Check baby's abdomen 10 to 20 minutes after a feeding. Milk that is easily digested and quickly empties from the tummy will not cause the abdomen to look and feel bloated. On the other hand, undigested milk that just sits there gives off gas, which inflates and irritates baby's sensitive intestines, leading to colicky abdominal pain and bloating. If baby's tummy feels and sounds like a drum after eating, slow down the feedings and offer smaller amounts more frequently. If the bloating doesn't improve, change formulas.

Explosive stools. When undigested milk reaches the lower intestines, baby's stools are affected. You will hear the bowel movement shoot out from his bottom into the diaper, and baby will fuss when this happens. Again, this may not be due to the type of formula. Explosive stools are a common sign of overfeeding (even in term babies). If too much goes in too fast at one end, it's going to come out too fast at the other end. Try giving smaller, slower, more frequent feedings before switching formulas.

Anal rash. Undigested milk becomes acidic in the lower intestines, which can cause a red, rough burnlike rash around the anal opening. We call this the target sign. The acid content of baby's stools irritates the skin. If this is the only sign of formula intolerance, the first thing to do is to apply a white diaper cream with zinc oxide to baby's bottom after diaper changes. This will keep the irritating stools from coming into contact with baby's sensitive skin. If a severe rash persists, change the formula.

Dr. Jim advises: Always consult your baby's doctor before changing formulas, since some formulas, especially soy-based formulas, may not be appropriate for your baby.

NIGHT FEEDINGS

Should I feed my baby during the night?

Yes. Your preemie was probably fed on a schedule throughout the night in the NICU. Continue doing so for a while at home. Your baby needs these overnight feedings for several reasons. If she isn't fed during the night, she will need larger feedings during the day, and her tiny preemie tummy may not tolerate these. Also, going without food for long stretches at night can lower blood sugar, and this can be a problem for preemies. Feeding at night will help your baby take in more calories and grow better. Expect your preemie to need a feeding every 3 to 4 hours during the night. As your baby gets older and starts sleeping longer at night, you will be able to cut back on nighttime feedings.

III

PARENTING YOUR PREEMIE AT HOME

Finally your baby is home. Even though you will miss all the expert help and support you had 24/7 in the NICU, it's nice to settle down into the roles of mother and father. In this section, we will help you prepare for baby's homecoming. We will give you tips on how to develop a style of parenting that not only meets the unique needs of your preemie but also helps you enjoy your baby more. You will also find information that will prepare you to manage the most common challenges of baby's first year. Finally, in chapter 12 we will discuss the most common medical challenges that preemies face. Enjoy your baby at home! You have all worked hard to get there.

Homecoming

THE COUNTDOWN BEGINS! The doctors have told you that baby will be going home in just a few days! Suddenly you realize that there's a lot you have to do to get ready.

By now you probably feel quite comfortable in the NICU, working with the nurses to care for your baby. True, for weeks you've been saying that you can't wait to get your baby home. But, you wonder, can you really care for your preemie all by yourself?

Your baby's needs are changing. That's why it is time to leave the hospital. Your baby will still need "intensive" care for a while, but now the special care he needs is more maternal than mechanical. The NICU gives way to the PICU — that's parent intensive care unit — which is infinitely more peaceful and personal. Whether you feel ready to bring your baby home or apprehensive about your ability to care for her (most likely you feel some of both), you are moving into a new stage of life with your preemie.

My baby's homecoming was both happy and sad. Sad because the medical staff had been our new extended family (she was a micropreemie at 25 weeks and in the NICU for 14 weeks), so it was hard to leave them; happy because our miracle baby was finally coming home.

PREPARING FOR D-DAY

The transition from NICU to home requires planning on many fronts. In the hospital, there may be last-minute details about baby's care for you to master. At home, you'll need preemie baby clothes, diapers, and other equipment, some unique to preemies. You need to get yourself ready for the job of full-time baby care. Keep in mind that while the doctors may have told you that you can expect to take baby home on such-and-such a date, anything can happen. Baby's homecoming may suddenly be postponed because of medical problems. Or you may get a surprise and discover that departure day is sooner than you expected. Here are some suggestions for getting ready for the big day.

Rest up. At least for a few days before the planned discharge, get as much rest and relaxation as you can so you will be at your best to care for your baby. A veteran NICU nurse in our local hospital suggests: "Mom and Dad should go out on a last date before baby comes home. It may be a while before they get to enjoy a night out together."

It helps to prepare ahead of time for those busy first few days at home.

Rehearse your role. Ask the nurses if you can be your baby's primary caregiver in the hospital for a day or two before you go home, with the nurses available to answer questions and provide reassurance. Pretend that you are at home and care for your baby from morning until night: feeding, diapering, bathing, positioning to sleep, and managing any medications or machinery that you might be using at home. Get an overall feel for what a day with your baby will be like at home. The NICU may have a special room for you, where you can stay overnight with your baby. Or you may prefer to go home at night and get some sleep while you can. While you have expert helpers close by, use this special day or two to gain confidence in your ability to take over baby's care. Ask for their help when you need it, but also try to relax and rely on your own knowledge of your baby to solve any problems that come up.

If any relatives or substitute caregivers are going to be taking care of baby, it is vital that they also receive teaching from the nurses while baby is still in the NICU.

Get some professional help. By now you've met the NICU social worker. He or she is a key helper as you plan for your baby's discharge from the hospital. While the nurses can answer your questions about your baby's personal and medical care, the social worker is your connection to services outside the hospital. He or she can arrange for equipment to be delivered to your home and refer you to sources for other supplies you may need. The social worker can also help you find the services you need in your community, such as an early intervention program that will monitor baby's development and provide physical or occupational therapy or speech and language therapy.

Prepare a homecoming checklist. Depending on your baby's special needs and what you have already done in anticipation of bringing baby home, your list may be long or short. You will have to take care of many of the items on your list personally, but other items can be delegated to friends and family members who have offered to help. Put the checklist in your journal, your handbag, or some other place where it will be readily available. You will want to make notes and add items to the list as they occur to you.

☐ *Medications.* Be sure you know what medications your baby will need at home, the dosage, when to give them, and how long your baby may need them. Practice giving medications under the supervision of the nurses in the hospital before baby's discharge.

You may want to prepare a spreadsheet with a schedule of times and doses.

☐ *Special equipment.* Inquire ahead of time about any equipment your baby is likely to need at home, such as an apnea monitor, oxygen, or scale. If you are taking baby home with an apnea monitor (see page 192), be sure you are well trained in its use. If your baby comes home needing extra oxygen, be sure you understand how and when it should be used, when the amount should be increased (when to "up his O_2"), how to adjust the pulse oxygen monitor, how to attach the nasal canula, and how often to change the canula. Also, the oxygen needs to be humidified, so be sure you understand how to use this equipment. The discharge planner (a nurse or the social worker) will help you order the equipment and learn how to use it. When the equipment is delivered to your home, the technician will explain how to work the various dials and connections on a particular machine, which may look a little different from the one you practiced on in the hospital.

☐ *Discharge summary.* Ask for a copy of your baby's discharge summary, a report on your baby's NICU treatment and medical concerns from the hospital doctors. Take this with you to baby's first appointment with your pediatrician. While the hospital will automatically send a copy of the discharge summary to your doctor, this may take several weeks. It's wise to bring your own copy to your first checkup with your pediatrician.

☐ *Feedings.* By the time baby is ready to leave the hospital, you will have had some practice with feedings. Be sure that you are familiar with the bottles, nipples, tubings, and supplements that worked best for your baby in the hospital. Ask to take some of these home with you and inquire about where you can conveniently purchase more.

☐ *Breastfeeding supplies.* Check your breast pump, milk-storage supplies, nursing supplementer, and whatever else you may need to continue breastfeeding your baby. You may have to continue pumping for a few weeks, until your baby completes the transition to feeding at the breast. Having an extra collection kit means you have to wash pump parts only half as often. Extra parts for your nursing supplementer may also come in handy. (If you purchase these items at the hospital, the cost may be covered by your insurance.)

☐ *Car seat.* Be sure you buy an approved car seat for your baby. Have it installed properly before baby's discharge. Your baby will look very tiny in the car seat. Fill in the space around her with rolled blankets or your baby sling. (See Car Travel, page 176.)

☐ *Clothing.* Naturally, most baby clothes will seem big initially, but you'll be surprised at how fast your baby will grow into them. By now you know which clothing is most comfortable for your baby and easiest for caregivers to manage. Stick with that same style at home. Larger retailers may carry clothes sized especially for preemies. Or check the Internet to shop without leaving home (see Resources, page 235). Because baby's skin is extra sensitive, choose clothing that is soft on the inside. Since sizes vary, buy a couple outfits and try them on baby in the hospital. Find out which ones work the best and then buy more. The good news about buying clothes for preemies is that everything will fit eventually — though nice toasty sleepers won't be much use if they're the right size only in the middle of a hot summer.

☐ *Receiving blankets.* You'll need a couple of these for the trips from the hospital to home and from home to various follow-up appointments. If you are bringing baby home in the middle of winter, you'll need a warm bunting or other outer garment that accommodates car seat straps, plus extra warm blankets.

☐ *Diapers.* Both disposable and cloth diapers are available in preemie sizes. Like with clothing, softness is the key. To avoid chafing around baby's middle, fold the disposable's polyurethane edge outward, so that only the softer lining touches baby's skin. Whether you use disposables or cloth is a matter of cost, convenience, the sensitivity of your baby's skin, and your own preference. Even if you use disposables for diapering, you'll want a generous supply of cloth diapers to use as burping cloths.

☐ *Sleeping equipment.* Give some thought to your baby's sleeping arrangement before you bring him home from the hospital. Prior to his homecoming, purchase a bassinet, an Arm's Reach Co-Sleeper (a baby bed with an open side that can be placed next to your mattress for sleep sharing), a crib, or an Amby Bed (see page 161). You may even decide to have baby sleep in your bed. (Be open to different sleeping arrangements in the weeks to come. Don't be tied down to a certain crib or bassinet if it isn't working.)

☐ *Phone numbers.* Be sure to get phone numbers for the NICU, your baby's neonatologist, your lactation consultant, and any doctors, therapists, clinics, or programs that will be following up on your baby's care. Don't forget to get the phone numbers or e-mail addresses of other parents who have become your friends in the NICU. Ask the nurses which number to use and what the best time to call is if you need their reassurance or advice. Ask the nurse who knows you and your baby best if it's all right to call her specifically if you have a question while you're settling in at home. NICU nurses expect these calls and are happy to oblige (they want to know how you're doing), but try not to overdo it. Before calling, make a written list of your questions and try to lump all your queries into a single call. Nurses have plenty to do every day in the NICU, and you need to learn to rely on your own caregiving abilities at home.

☐ *Follow-up appointments.* Be sure you understand whom to see and when: baby's pediatrician, the ophthalmologist (if a follow-up eye exam is advised), other medical specialists, the preemie follow-up clinic, and early intervention services. Your nurse or social worker will help you get hooked up with all the services you need. You might want to make the necessary appointments before you leave the hospital, during one of those inevitable boring waiting periods. You'll have other things to worry about when you get home.

☐ *CPR class*. Be sure you have completed your CPR class and feel both knowledgeable and competent. If you will have regular substitute caregivers at home, be sure they take the CPR class, too. Get your CPR questions answered before leaving the hospital. (See Newborn and Infant CPR, page 225.)

FEELINGS YOU MAY HAVE

While you're happy that your preemie is healthy enough to come home, naturally this transition brings with it new feelings — both positive and negative.

Relieved. Finally you're home — and with your baby! When you wake up in the morning, you won't have to drive to the hospital. Baby will be right there, next to you. (In fact, baby may be what woke you up!) In many ways, preemie parents are better prepared for those first days at home than parents of full-term babies, who typically come home from the hospital a day or two after delivery. You have already had weeks, or sometimes months, to get to know your baby in the hospital before coming home with her. Parents of term infants often spend

weeks adjusting to their baby's unique needs and quirks.

One day when I was changing her diaper, I realized she had a bum. Previously her bottom had just been skin and bones — literally. There was no fat there! Once I noticed she had two tiny cheeks on her bottom, I gave them a gentle pat. That became my ritual day after day. Every time I finished changing her diaper, I gave her a soft squeeze on her bottom because finally she had one.

Anxious. Surprisingly, it may take time to get accustomed to the more flexible schedule of life at home after so many weeks of hospital routines. It takes time to relax into your new life. You may feel a bit anxious without the nurses around and without the monitors to reassure you that baby's heartbeat and breathing are normal. You may even find yourself wondering when someone from food services will bring your lunch tray. Home is bound to be different from the NICU. No matter how much you've looked forward to caring for your baby in the privacy of your own home, it will seem strange at first.

For a while, I found I was automatically taking my baby's temperature prior to changing his diaper because that's what I did in the hospital. It's hard to let go of the hospital routines and follow your parental instincts. It takes a while to phase out of the routines you learned in the NICU.

Tired. In the hospital, you could count on the nurses to be substitute caregivers when you went out for a walk or home to sleep. At home, you and your partner are in charge of baby 24/7. Expect your baby to wake up to be fed every couple hours day and night. Welcome to the tired world of parenting babies, where parents should try to grab a nap at every opportunity.

We thought we were bringing home a happy baby who would eat six to eight times a day and sleep a lot at night. She ended up eating ten to fourteen times a day and sleeping very little. We were very unprepared for this.

Protective. You will automatically be overprotective of your special baby, and this is perfectly appropriate. Friends and family may want you to relax and not worry so much, but you need to do this at your own pace. After you spent weeks witnessing how much extra care and monitoring your baby needed in the hospital, it's normal to continue that heightened watchfulness at home. After a few weeks' experience successfully caring for your baby by yourself, you will find that you are easing up on the constant surveillance.

I admit that sometimes I used to poke my sleeping baby just to make sure she was still breathing.

Home alone. At times, you will enjoy being home alone with your baby, but at other times, you may miss the NICU staff and the company of the other preemie parents. Many mothers are not prepared for how isolated they feel at home with baby. You may not want to go out in public because of the risk of exposing your baby to germs or the challenge of lugging around an apnea monitor (see Going Home with an Apnea Monitor, page 192, for how to travel with a monitor). When you want to connect with other adults,

use the phone. Call one of the mothers you met in the NICU, or plan to talk to a supportive friend or family member several times a week. The Internet is another way to connect with people — even at 2 a.m. You may want to explore bulletin boards, chat rooms, or e-mail lists for parents of preemies. You can also use e-mail to let friends and family know how you and baby are doing, in both words and pictures.

I became somewhat of a recluse for a while, staying home all the time and not wanting anyone to come over. In part, I was afraid of germs, but really I felt like I needed a month alone with my son for every day we had to leave the hospital without him. I am truly grateful that I was able to make up for some of the lost bonding time.

Dr. Bob advises: You and baby don't need to be housebound. As long as the weather is not too cold and there are no medical reasons for keeping baby inside, you and baby can take daily walks. Wear your baby in a sling and walk around the neighborhood. The sling will help keep baby warm and settled and discourage neighbors and passersby from peering at and touching baby. Babies oftentimes have fussy periods toward the end of the day (moms and dads do, too). We call this the "happy hour." It is a good time to put your fussy baby in a sling and take a walk. You'll both feel better.

MAKING A HOME FOR YOUR BABY

While your baby was in the NICU, her environment was well regulated. She was kept warm, she was fed and changed routinely, and daily weight checks and frequent vital sign assessments confirmed that everything was going well. Experienced nurses responded to her cues and kept her from getting overstimulated. Now that you are bringing her home, it is going to be up to you to shape her environment. Of course, the most important feature of her environment is you — your loving arms, your warm skin, your willingness to care for her night and day. But there are several other aspects of your baby's home environment that deserve your attention, too.

Peace and quiet. Despite the occasional beeping alarms and hectic activity during medical emergencies, most NICUs are relatively quiet. It's important for you to continue this tranquil atmosphere at home for the next few weeks, until your baby adjusts to more stimulating surroundings. Instruct other family members at home to be careful not to upset baby with too much noise and activity. Yet, you don't have to be perfectly quiet around baby. Sounds of everyday life are unavoidable at home. There's no need to make everyone "tiptoe and hush" around baby all day long. It's okay to make some noise, to talk, laugh, and play near baby, as long as the volume is kept to a reasonable level. Let your other kids be kids. Avoid sudden loud noises, such as kitchen appliances, vacuum cleaners, shouting, and loud music. While older children have been waiting a long time to play with baby, remind them to be gentle and to speak softly. Limit the length of your preemie's playtime; preemies need to rest and sleep in order to grow.

Stable temperature. Your baby is able to regulate and maintain his body tempera-

ture reasonably well; otherwise he wouldn't be at home with you. You don't need to be overly careful about room temperatures, but it is better to avoid extremes. A comfortable 65 to 80° F is best for baby. You don't necessarily need to measure baby's temperature at home (unless the NICU staff has instructed you to). You know your baby is at a comfortable temperature if his hands and feet are warm and his head is not sweating. If baby's head is sweaty, then you know he's too warm, and it may be time to take off a layer of his clothing. If his hands and feet are cold, then he needs a warmer outfit or a blanket. Keeping baby close to you in a sling will help keep him warm even if it's winter and your house is drafty.

Germ-free environment. Remember all the hand washing you did in the NICU? Well, don't lose this habit just yet. Remember to wash your hands after using the bathroom, blowing your nose, going outside, coming home from work, or running errands. Insist that your other children wash their hands as well. However, you must also realize that you, your baby, and your other family members are going to share germs. Your baby was certainly exposed to some germs in the NICU, and he will be exposed to germs at home, no matter how careful you are. You don't need to wash your hands every hour, or every time you go to touch your baby. Immediate family should also be free to touch and hold the baby without first being "sterilized."

When baby's siblings or other immediate family members are sick with colds or other "bugs," do the best you can to keep them from physical contact with your preemie — no kissing or sticking fingers in baby's mouth. If your baby is breastfeeding, your milk will help to protect him from the common germs to which both of you are exposed in your home.

Avoid group care like the plague. Don't leave your baby in day care or in the nursery at church or the fitness center until he is 6 months of age, and even longer if you are able. Leaving your baby among other infants, toddlers, and preschoolers for even an hour is asking for a cold, flu, or diarrhea illness. Premature babies are especially susceptible to cold viruses, and what might be a minor cold or flu in an older child or adult can turn into a serious respiratory infection in a preemie.

Crowd control. All those neighbors and relatives who've been longing to see your little baby but couldn't visit the NICU are now going to be knocking on your door. You may wish to limit visitors for a few weeks while you are settling into making a home for your baby. When you want to open your home to welcomed visitors, be aware that every person who walks through your door will be accompanied by millions of germs. You should insist on thorough hand washing for any visitor who steps into your house. Before letting visitors come over to see your baby, be certain they are completely well. Be straightforward and thorough in your questions. Don't worry about hurt feelings — you have a baby to protect and keep well. When you explain that even the slightest cold can be hazardous to your baby, the people who care about your family will understand.

Fresh air. Go ahead and take your baby outside for daily walks (in good weather of course). Going outside won't make your baby catch a cold. It's being around sick people that will make your baby sick. When you do take baby to gatherings of friends and relatives, don't be timid about keeping baby close to you. Passing a preemie around to a dozen friends is asking for an illness. Keep your baby snuggled in a sling and tucked into a blanket. This will help ward off curious hands.

Swaddling. Your baby may be accustomed to always being swaddled up tight in the NICU. While it's okay to swaddle baby for a nap from time to time, her legs and arms also need to stretch and move around. Give baby time every day to exercise those limbs. Keeping baby's legs constantly wrapped up tightly in the "burrito position" can be detrimental to her hip development.

Dr. Jim advises: Try to make a *home* for your baby, not just an extension of the hospital.

SETTING UP YOUR TEAM OF HELPERS

While your baby was in the NICU, you probably counted on support from family and friends. They may have brought meals to your home and entertained your other kids. Now that baby is coming home, you need this kind of support more than ever. Parents of full-term newborns enjoy this kind of pampering from sisters, aunts, and grandmas during the early postpartum period. You deserve it now. Don't be afraid to ask for help. Don't be too proud to admit that you need it. Even if you don't feel like you need help, realize that every little favor from a friend means one fewer task you have to do that day. You can take the time you save and lavish it on your baby, or, just as important, on yourself. Here is a list of favors your family and friends can do for you. All you have to do is ask.

☐ *Meals.* Nothing helps you enjoy your baby more than knowing that dinner is already cooked and ready to go. Few things are as satisfying as a homemade meal, with a nice salad and cooked vegetables. Perhaps a friend could call up all the people who have offered their help and put together a schedule for bringing meals to your family. Casseroles are probably the easiest — everything is in one dish. All you do (or Dad does) is heat and serve. An already-mixed salad makes it a complete meal. The leftovers can be lunch tomorrow, or you can stash them in the freezer for next week.

☐ *Wheels.* Do you have errands to run? Clothes to take to the cleaners? Mail for the post office? Kids to take to school or soccer practice? Need groceries? Put away your car keys for a couple weeks and ask others to run your errands along with theirs.

☐ *Housework.* Are the dirty clothes piling up? The dishes dirty? Dust bunnies running wild? Ask each visitor to complete one or two simple tasks.

☐ *Babysitting.* If you have other kids, get a babysitter once or twice a month so that you and your husband can go out for a quiet dinner. Take baby with you if you wish, while he's still willing to sleep through much of dinner. Or leave him at home if that's what you need to do to enjoy an hour or two to yourselves.

☐ *Baby holding.* Need to grab a nice uninterrupted nap? Let someone else hold the baby for an hour or two while you catch up on sleep. Or you may prefer to get some things done around the house that only you can do. A grandma who has been itching to hold the baby is perfect for this job.

☐ *"No" is never an answer.* People are going to ask you almost every day, "Is there anything I can do for you?" Resist the temptation to say, "No, I'm doing fine." Say yes!

☐ *Price of admission.* A creative way to ask for help is to "charge admission" to your house for the baby show. Ask anyone who calls up and wants to come over to bring a meal or stop by the grocery store.

HANDLING SIBLINGS

Whenever a new baby arrives, parents naturally worry about how their older kids will adjust. Siblings' reactions to the new family member depend mostly upon their age. Children four years and older are usually very excited about a new baby, and any jealous feelings are minimal, whereas two- and three-year-olds often have mixed feelings about a new baby.

Besides the age-old problem of jealousy between siblings, bringing home a premature baby may create other kinds of stress for your kids. Older children may worry about the baby's health, express more concern over baby's day-to-day well-being, and even fear that baby will have to go

PROTECTING BABY'S PRECIOUS LUNGS

Because the lungs are one of the most fragile and problematic systems in preemies, they require special care. Here are some guidelines for making your home a lung-friendly environment:

No smoking, please! Smoking around baby not only irritates the already fragile lining of baby's breathing passages but also greatly increases the risk of Sudden Infant Death Syndrome. Exposure to smoke can increase the risk of SIDS as much as fivefold. Also, children of parents who smoke have two to three times more doctor visits because of respiratory infections.

Breathing passages are lined with tiny filaments called cilia, which wave back and forth to clear mucus from the airway. Smoke paralyzes these cilia, allowing mucus to clog the air passages. When colds or allergies cause the body to secrete more mucus than usual, the bad effects of smoking on baby's breathing increase.

Mothers who smoke have lower levels of prolactin, the hormone that regulates milk production and may contribute to intuitive mothering. Studies have shown that mothers who smoke do not breastfeed as long as mothers who don't, perhaps because of problems with milk supply.

Minimize exposure to germs. Avoid putting your preemie in group day care as much as possible, especially during fall and winter. This is when RSV (the respiratory syncytial virus) runs rampant among infants (see page 186 for a description of this serious lung disease). Any baby who spends any time at all, even as little as an hour a week, in a nursery setting is almost sure to be exposed to RSV. If day care is unavoidable, an in-home setting where one caregiver cares for only a few children is safer than an environment that exposes your baby to a larger group of infants and toddlers. (Besides RSV, com-

---

back into the hospital. Toddlers may resent the new baby not only because of the time you spend caring for your preemie now, but also because of the hours and hours you were away from home while baby was in the NICU. Here are some suggestions that may help your other children to cope with their fears and jealousy:

Model peace and a positive attitude. If you maintain a positive outlook, your kids will pick up on this. If they sense you are not worried, they won't be either. Remem-

ber, your kids can read you better than you think. You can't easily turn that positive attitude off and on. If they hear you fretting over possible complications with your preemie, they too will begin to fear that something might go wrong with the baby. Not only will they worry about their sibling, but they'll know that if baby has to go back to the hospital, this will take you away from them again. Anxiety in children can cause physical symptoms, such as stomachaches and headaches, and can worsen behavior problems. Give them mon cold, flu, and diarrhea-causing viruses are also prevalent in day care situations.)

Protect your baby from RSV. Check to see if your baby meets the guidelines for RSV preventive medicine (see page 187). If so, follow the monthly schedule to protect your baby from this serious respiratory infection.

Allergy-proof baby's room. Get rid of objects that are magnets for mold or dust, such as fuzzy toys and piles of clothing or books. For tips on allergy proofing baby's bedroom, consult www.AskDrSears.com/allergies.

Make room air more lung friendly. Moisture in the air makes it easier for babies to breathe. The humidity helps keep the normal secretions of the respiratory passages moist, preventing clogged-up noses and irritated throats.

So, don't think only of the temperature of the air in your home, consider the humidity as well. Babies' lungs are happiest with humidity around 50 percent. Higher humidity levels encourage the growth of allergens such as mold; lower levels can dry out baby's sensitive breathing passages. In cold climates, central heating can drastically lower the humidity of room air, but it's easy to remedy the situation. A simple hot-mist vaporizer will keep the air in a small bedroom comfortably warm and moist. Be sure to place the vaporizer out of the reach of baby and other small children and to change the filter regularly. Hide the cord behind a dresser so that a toddler can't pull the whole thing down with a yank on the electrical cord. Humidifying the air stabilizes the temperature in the room — a perk for preemies with unstable body temperatures.

an "everything's all right" atmosphere. This will also help to lessen your own anxiety.

Talk honestly with older kids. You must decide how much your kids can understand and how much to share with them. If your baby is completely healthy, with no medical problems as a result of prematurity, then be sure to emphasize this to your kids. If your baby does have some ongoing concerns, you don't need to explain these in great detail to your kids, but

you do need to talk about them. Give them simple answers to their questions, but don't try to evade the issue or they may worry that you are keeping something from them. Whatever they imagine is wrong is probably much scarier than the truth.

Involve your kids with baby's care. One sure way to minimize your toddler's jealousy is to keep him close to you and baby. Constantly talk to your toddler while feeding or changing the baby. Ask for your toddler to hand you a new diaper or baby wipe, to hold baby's hand, or to help with bath time. But be careful that your toddler doesn't feel that all you ever do together is take care of baby. Find things you can do with your toddler while you feed or hold the baby, such as reading a book or playing a quiet game.

Handle with care, but not too much.
Parents of preemies handle their babies with extra care and tenderness. When siblings want to hold or play with the baby, parents may try to discourage them for fear that the new baby is too fragile. Picture for a moment what your toddler is thinking: "Here is a new baby that Mom keeps to herself all the time." If you always say "no" or "be careful" or "don't touch the baby," your toddler will definitely grow to resent the new sib. She wants to interact with that baby, and if she can't do it with your help, she'll find her own angry ways of making contact.

Allow your toddler to interact with the baby in a way that is safe. Let her kiss baby, hug baby, rub baby's tummy, pat baby's back, and play with baby's hands and feet. Instead of saying no, show her how to love baby safely and gently. Teach her ways to play that will not overstimulate baby.

FIRST VISIT TO BABY'S DOCTOR

Most pediatricians have experience in caring for premature babies. You don't need to look for a special doctor for your baby. If you selected a pediatrician while you were pregnant or if you already have a pediatrician for your older children, this will probably be the doctor you choose to care for your preemie. He or she will help you monitor baby's weight gain and feeding patterns and observe baby closely for any medical or developmental problems. If you are planning to breastfeed long term, be sure to find a breastfeeding-friendly pediatrician who will support you, preferably one with a lactation consultant on staff. Having a supportive doctor and medical staff will be invaluable to you in continuing your breastfeeding relationship with your baby.

Here is a checklist of items that your pediatrician will want to see at your first visit:

☐ *Discharge summary from the NICU.* Before leaving the NICU, ask the doctor or nurse to give you a summary of your baby's care so far, including copies of important test results, a list of medications, and notes on medical problems that need ongoing attention. The NICU doctor will also create a dictated summary of baby's care for the hospital record, but completing this can take weeks. It won't be ready for your first visit with the pediatrician.

☐ *Baby's weight at the time of discharge.* Your pediatrician will want to know how much your baby weighed when you left the hospital. Also, if your baby has been weighed by a visiting nurse or anyone else since leaving the NICU, be sure to write that information down, with the date, and give it to your pediatrician.

☐ *Feeding, pooping, and peeing diary.* Keep a record of what goes in and what comes out and bring this to your first appointment. (If you're breastfeeding and can't measure how much milk is going in, make some notes about how often your baby feeds, for how long, and how effectively he seems to nurse.) Your record gives the doctor useful information about how things are going at home.

☐ *Written list of questions.* Write down any questions that come up while at home.

☐ *Bring any medications you are giving baby to your office visit.* This way, your doctor can know exactly what medications, if any, your baby is taking.

☐ *Bring along your journal.* Continue your baby's progress and "grow journal" you kept in the hospital. This can also be a good place to write down your questions as they occur to you. Review the journal in the waiting room. Afterward, jot down memorable notes from your doctor visits.

IMMUNIZATIONS BEFORE DISCHARGE

Before baby leaves the NICU, he may get one or more of the following routine childhood vaccines, just like a full-term 2-month-old infant would:

Hepatitis B. This is a blood-borne illness that damages the liver.

DTaP. Diphtheria, tetanus, and pertussis are serious childhood diseases.

Haemophilus influenza type b. This is a bacteria that causes meningitis.

Polio. This is a potentially paralyzing disease.

Pneumococcus. This bacteria causes pneumonia and meningitis.

Depending on your baby's age at discharge, he may get some or all of these shots. Your pediatrician will continue these throughout the year.

Developing a Parenting Style That's Best for Preemies

SUPPOSE YOUR DOCTOR could prescribe a pill that could help your preemie grow faster, healthier, and smarter, lessen the chances and severity of medical problems preemies are prone to, and boost your confidence as a parent. Of course you would eagerly give your baby such medicine. Guess what? There is such a "pill," and you don't even need a prescription for it. This "medicine" is called attachment parenting (AP).

In the days after your preemie's birth, you may have worried about whether you were up to the challenge of being the parent of a tiny baby with such intense needs. You'll leave the hospital with plenty of instructions about caring for your baby and visiting doctors for follow-up care, but how will you know what to do when the baby cries or won't go to sleep or wakes up in the middle of the night? And how will *you* survive the worrying and the hard work of caring for your baby?

We have an answer to all these questions: practice attachment parenting. Preemie babies are indeed special babies who

need a special kind of parenting to help them achieve their full potential. Attachment parenting is a style of infant care that brings out the best in babies and their parents. The tools of AP help you meet the special needs of your special baby. While AP benefits all babies, it's particularly useful for preemies and their parents.

The attachment strategies you advise are helpful for all parents, but they are essential for preemie parents.

THE SEVEN BABY B'S

The tools of attachment parenting are ways of interacting with and caring for your baby that help you and your child get connected. We call these tools the Baby B's, and they have special importance to parents caring for premature babies. Depending on the medical condition of your baby and your family's lifestyle, you may not be able to practice all of the Baby B's all of the time. Practice as many as you can with the resources you have.

ATTACHMENT PARENTING — BABY'S BEST RX	
Problems Preemies May Have	**How AP Helps**
• breathing difficulties • delayed motor development • delayed cognitive development • difficulties with attention • restless sleep patterns • susceptibility to infections • delayed growth • behavioral problems • digestive problems (e.g., reflux) • tendency to be fussy and easily startled	• regulates breathing • improves motor development • improves cognitive development (i.e., makes babies smarter) • helps babies focus • promotes restful sleep • boosts immunity • accelerates growth • improves behavior • improves digestion • promotes calmness and security
Problems Parents May Have	**How AP Helps**
• postpartum depression • difficulty reading baby's cues • lack of connection to baby • confusion about what baby needs • anxiety about baby, lack of confidence	• lessens postpartum depression • helps you read baby's cues • helps you feel connected • helps you be more sensitive and responsive to baby's needs • helps you feel confident

1. Birth Bonding

Bonding obviously takes on a different meaning when prematurity makes it impossible for parents to hold their baby in their arms in the hours immediately after birth. It's important for parents of preemies to take advantage of other ways of nourishing their attachment to their baby. These include staying close to baby in the early hours and days after his birth, getting involved with his care, touching him in the isolette, and eventually holding him when he is ready to tolerate this kind of stimulation. Kangaroo care is a wonderful substitute for birth bonding. In fact, it's much the same thing, including, as it does, peaceful skin-to-skin contact, baby's first explorations of mother's nipple, and attachment hormones flowing through mother's veins. (One of the pioneers of kangaroo care, Dr. Nils Bergman, has suggested that all newborns — full-term and premature — need kangaroo care, since mother's body is their "natural habitat," and removing them to other environments, such as a crib, is stressful.) How soon and how much K care you are able to practice with your baby depends a lot on the medical condition of your baby and the hospital's policies, but do take advantage of every opportunity to be in touch with your baby!

2. Breastfeeding

As you learned in detail in chapter 6, mother's milk is the best medicine for premature infants. Now that your baby is ready to go home, breastfeeding's benefits for your baby become even greater. Breastfeeding will help you learn to interpret and respond to baby's signals. Because breastfeeding is an exercise in baby reading, it helps you more intuitively read baby's cues for care and feeding, which may be more subtle than the cues of a term baby. It ensures that you spend a lot of time focusing on your baby. It guarantees that you get a chance to sit down and relax many times each day. Pumping and storing your milk in the days after baby's birth was a lot of work, and teaching baby to nurse at the breast may have been challenging as well. Yet in the days to come, as baby gets stronger and able to help himself at "Mom's diner," you'll find that breastfeeding is convenient, rewarding, and fun! Enjoy it!

3. Babywearing

As we talk to parents shortly before baby is discharged from the hospital, one of the "doctor's orders" we share with them is this: "Wear your baby in a baby sling at least three hours a day." While baby is still in the hospital, or during the family's first visit to our office, we give parents and their preemie a "sling demo" to acquaint them with the art of babywearing. In our view, babywearing should be part of standard preemie care, just like feeding and changing diapers.

Babywearing is certainly nothing new. Carrying baby on mother's body or on the

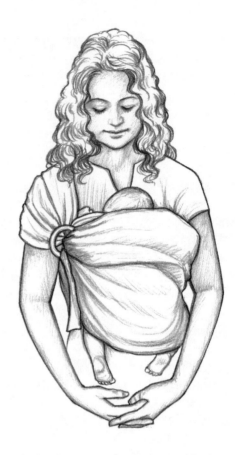

body of another adult caregiver is as natural a part of human infant care as breastfeeding. Human babies need constant protection, and a mother's instinct is to keep baby in her arms, close to her. The closeness is rewarding for both mother and baby and builds the attachment between them. (See www.AskDrSears.com/babywearing for step-by-step instructions on how to wear a newborn in a baby sling.) While all babies benefit from babywearing, preemies benefit even more. We advise every parent of a preemie to raise a "sling baby." Here's why:

Sling babies cry less. Crying is not good for babies, especially preemies. It wastes

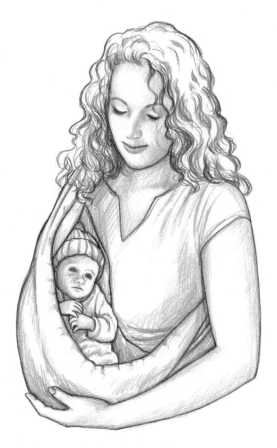

This stimulation helps baby feel peaceful. Babywearing reminds baby of the motion and secure balance he enjoyed in the womb. Baby got used to the rhythm of mother's walk while in the womb, and he now experiences this familiar rhythm in the "outside womb" during babywearing.

Realize your baby will need "more" because she missed out on a lot of womb time. Wear your baby a lot. Sometimes it's the only way to keep baby happy while you get things done around the house.

Sling babies breathe better. Moving in three dimensions stimulates babies' vestibular system, the part of the nervous system that controls balance, and research has shown that vestibular stimulation helps preemies breathe and grow better. The vestibular system relies on three tiny balance centers in the inner ear that work like carpenter's levels, one tracking side-to-side motion, another for up-and-down motion, and a third for back-and-forth motion. They all function together to keep the body in balance. Every time you move, the fluid in these "levels" comes into contact with tiny hairlike filaments that vibrate and send messages to the brain. The brain uses the information to keep you from toppling over.

While baby is in the watery environment of the womb, baby's vestibular system is constantly stimulated by mother's movement. After birth, babies seem to expect this gentle motion to continue. Studies of premature babies placed on oscillating water beds showed that they not only grew better but had fewer apnea episodes. Smart little babies recognize they need vestibular stimulation. Infants

oxygen and energy that preemies need for catch-up growth. A research study has shown that infants who were carried an extra three hours a day cried and fussed 43 percent less than infants whose parents were not advised to give them extra carrying time.

Research has shown that it's not only the amount of time baby is carried that reduces crying time, it's also the way baby is held. When baby is worn in a sling, baby moves gently in all possible directions (up and down, from side to side, and back and forth). Research has shown that babies cry less when they are moved in three dimensions of motion rather than just being rocked back and forth or from side to side.

who are deprived of adequate vestibular stimulation, those who are not rocked or carried often, frequently attempt to stimulate themselves with self-rocking movements. Preemies are especially prone to wasting energy in random movements. Babywearing provides the motion that helps babies' immature body system work better. Babies conserve energy when they don't have to provide this motion for themselves.

Dr. Bill says: Lots of good things happen physiologically when baby is nestled in a carrier close to a caregiver's body. I loved draping our babies skin-to-skin over my chest with their ear over my heartbeat. Also, while wearing our own babies, I noticed my breathing stimulated theirs. When I wore our sixth child, Matthew, in the sling and he slept nestled against my chest, I noticed that whenever I took a deep breath, so did he. Sometimes, when the air exhaled from my mouth and nose moved over his scalp, he would take a deep breath. (Martha and I dubbed this "magic breath.")

The connection between babywearing and babies' thriving has been known for a long time. Years ago I had the opportunity to interview parents from third world countries at an international parenting conference. I noticed these mothers were wearing their babies in various kinds of slings, many of which were made of fabric that matched their native dress. When I asked them why they carried their babies, I got very simple, but profound, answers, such as, "They cry less and they grow better." Keen observation through the centuries has taught mothers that babies thrive better when carried in slings. Modern researchers are just now confirming what mothers have known all along: babies do better when nestled close to a caregiver's body.

Sling babies feed better. This benefit of babywearing is a no-brainer. Wear a growing baby inches away from his favorite food source, and naturally he's going to, shall we say, visit the restaurant often. Proximity encourages frequent feeding, and the shorter the intervals between breastfeedings, the higher the fat content of a mother's milk. In a nutshell, frequent feedings encourage Mom to make more "grow milk." The two Baby B's of babywearing and breastfeeding naturally fit together.

Sling babies are smarter. Babies learn a lot in the arms of a busy caregiver. While motion calms babies, it doesn't necessarily put them to sleep. Babywearing promotes a state called quiet alertness, a behavioral

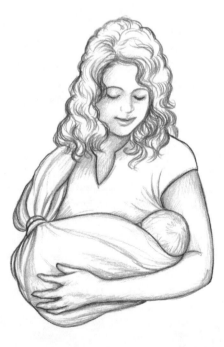

state in which babies are calm and can concentrate better and learn more. This is particularly important for preemies, since one of the long-term complications associated with prematurity is an increased incidence of problems paying attention and focusing. Infant developmental specialists feel that babies' physiological systems are more in balance in the state of quiet alertness, so they have more energy for interacting with caregivers and the environment.

Sling babies sleep better. Preemies tend to be restless sleepers. They squirm, startle, and awaken frequently. Over many years in pediatric practice, we have noticed that babies who are carried more during the day tend to have more restful nights. This is likely a result of the overall physiological regulation that babywearing promotes. The simple explanation is that babies get so used to being content during the day that they remain calm and restful at night.

Growing better, breathing better, feeding better, sleeping better, and thinking better all are a result of the simple pleasures of babywearing. Could this basic baby care tool do anything more? Read on.

Babywearing helps mothers and fathers, too! Parents of premature babies report two main concerns during the early months of parenting their preemies: a difficulty getting attached after being separated for so long, and a difficulty reading baby's cues. Babywearing helps parents with both of these challenges. When you wear baby for several hours a day "right under your nose," you spend a lot of time in eye-to-eye, face-to-face contact. You quickly learn to read baby's body and facial language and relate these specific movements and expressions to specific needs. Proximity promotes familiarity. A babywearing mother, for example, will often immediately sense that her baby is getting overstimulated by the way he squirms or grimaces. And because she and baby are right next to each other, she can immediately calm him *before baby fusses.* Baby doesn't have to go all the way into sensory overload before getting assistance from Mom. Minimizing a premature baby's fussing and crying time conserves his energy and promotes his growth. Even more important, it makes it easier for you to enjoy your baby.

WORDS TO FORGET

Some unfortunate words and phrases have crept into the vocabulary of parenting advice over the years. We try to keep these out of our writing, unless we're explaining why you should be forgetting them. They don't belong in the vocabulary of parents of term babies and definitely have no place in parenting premature babies:

- "cry it out" — don't let baby do this! (for reasons, see page 155)
- "colic" — a term we don't use for preemies (for reasons, see page 196)
- "spoil" — you can't spoil a tiny baby
- "manipulation" — babies are smart, but they're not devious
- "by now, baby should be . . ." — preemies have their own timetable; continuing to make progress is more important than reaching goals at a specific time

4. Belief in the Signal Value of Baby's Cry

A baby's cry is a baby's language, designed for the survival of the baby and the development of the mother. Listen to it. The general immaturity of preemies' central nervous system can cause them to fuss and cry more, yet because of their immature lungs, prolonged crying is very stressful for them physiologically. Adults react emotionally to babies' cries — nature designed the caregiving system that way, so that babies would get the attention they need. Try these cry mellowers:

Create conditions that reduce baby's need to cry. All the Baby B's of attachment parenting lessen a baby's need to cry. AP shapes baby's environment (you!) so that baby is mostly calm and content and doesn't need to cry to get her needs met. Carried babies cry less, breastfeeding babies are fed and held more, so they cry less, and bed-sharing infants (see below) cry less because Mom is right there.

My baby seldom cries; she doesn't need to.

Anticipate baby's precry signals. Studies show that the more quickly and consistently parents respond to baby's cries, the less baby cries in the long run. Notice baby's precry signals, such as grimacing, excited breathing, quivering lips, flailing arms, and a squirming body — all signs that something is not right. Getting to baby quickly and calming him down before the cry erupts is particularly important for anxious babies whose opening whimpers immediately escalate into frantic screaming. These babies are difficult to calm once they start crying, so a wise parent will do everything possible to respond to precry signals.

Respond quickly. It stands to reason that if you let your baby continue crying, he will learn that he has to settle himself on his own and eventually he will cry less. Right? Wrong. Studies of infant crying show the opposite to be true. Babies whose cries are promptly attended to gradually learn to cry less. Here's a basic parenting principle that applies to children from tiny newborns to teens: get behind the eyes of your child and imagine things from her viewpoint. When baby cries and no one comes to help, she feels helpless, insignificant, frightened, and alone. She really does not know how to calm herself. (She doesn't even know what it means to have a "self.") At this tender age, she's not going to learn to "pull herself up by her own bootstraps." She learns instead that she is powerless, that her cries have no effect whatsoever on her caregivers.

When you don't respond to your baby's cries, the two of you are in a lose-lose situation: baby loses trust in the signal value of his cries, and you lose the opportunity to become more sensitive to your baby. When you go against your instinct to respond to your baby's cries, you are shutting down a way of connecting with your child. Babies with persistent personalities may cry more loudly and harder when no one responds, and they may eventually get the response they are seeking, but they learn that the best way to get Mom's attention is to cry as hard and as loudly as they can. Other babies shut down after a while when no one responds to their cries. They may become very wary about trusting their environment.

Each crying episode is a cry-by-cry call. As you and your baby grow together, you will learn which cries need immediate attention and when baby can wait for a moment or two. Cry research reveals that a cry has two different phases: the early phase, in the first seconds, and the avoidance phase. The early phase is an attachment-promoting sound, which triggers a warm and empathetic response in the listener. If the early phase is not appropriately attended to, baby then enters the avoidance phase of the cry, which is more disturbing and irritating to the listener and often does not evoke an empathetic response. It is much harder to comfort baby once the cry enters this phase.

Keep on trying. You won't always know how to respond to baby's cries, and you won't always be able to comfort baby quickly. It's important that you do your best to minimize how often and how long your baby cries, but remember that it's not your fault that baby cries. Stay calm, and don't take it personally. The most important thing is that you just hang in there with your baby when he is fussy and upset. Do what you can to comfort and soothe him, but keep in mind that you can't "make" a baby stop crying.

5. Bedding Close to Baby

The Baby B that is the most controversial part of AP — and one of the most important — is bedding close to baby (also called cosleeping, sharing sleep, or, according to the older term, the family bed). Before you take baby home from the hospital, you need to think about where baby will sleep. We recommend that baby sleep *in whatever place makes it possible for all family members to sleep well.* This may well mean that baby shares sleep with

---

"CRY IT OUT" — NOT FOR PREEMIES

Once you have a baby, detach yourself from advice that detaches you from baby. Advisors will tell you, "Let your baby cry it out." We say, "Don't do it! And double-don't for preemies." Someone may say, "Crying is good for his lungs." We say, "It's not!" Excessive crying lowers a baby's blood oxygen level, which is already marginal in preemies. Even term infants and toddlers can "turn blue" from excessive crying. Don't let this happen to your preemie.

Here's how prolonged crying can lower a baby's blood oxygen. The sound of crying is caused by exhaling air against mostly closed vocal cords. When baby is crying, all of baby's energy goes into exhaling, and less air is inhaled. This means less oxygen gets into the blood. Also, the higher pressure generated in the chest cavity during a frantic cry can affect blood flow through the heart. Blood that has not yet been pumped to the lungs to pick up new oxygen may get diverted back out into the body. A preemie's brain and other vital organs will receive less oxygen during prolonged crying. The increased pressure in the abdomen that is associated with crying may also lead to spitting up or reflux, which preemies are already prone to. In short, crying wastes energy, wastes oxygen, and wastes food — all of which preemies need more of.

Mom and Dad. Consider these preemie perks of cosleeping.

Sleeping close to their mommies has unique physiological benefits for preemies. As you have learned, the central nervous system, the cardiorespiratory system, and the digestive system are all immature in preemies, and being physically close to mother helps these systems mature more quickly. Sharing sleep with mother helps preemies with catch-up growth and lessens breathing difficulties. Because preemies need to be fed more frequently, they naturally awaken more frequently. Expect the blissful "sleeping through the night" to be many months away. So it's necessary to work out a sleeping arrangement that enables you to feed your baby at night while still getting enough rest for yourself. Here's why this Baby B is good for parents and their preemies:

Babies — and mothers — sleep better. "But how will I sleep with baby right there next to me?" you may worry. Actually, once mother and baby get into "sleep harmony," most cosleeping mothers report sleeping better. Your milk contains natural sleep-inducing proteins, which help baby sleep. Baby's sucking stimulates the release of the hormone prolactin, which acts as a natural tranquilizer and helps you sleep. Both members of the nursing pair sleep better when they do what comes naturally.

Besides, sharing sleep with baby is much less disruptive to a mother's rest than being awakened by distant crying and then having to get out of a nice warm bed to rush down the hall to feed a hungry, frantic baby. By the time baby is fed and once again sleeping, Mom is wide awake and may not go back to sleep easily. Contrast this with a baby who awakens right next

to his mother. Mom senses from baby's movements that baby is restless and offers the breast. Baby nurses back to sleep, and Mom, who has barely awakened, also drifts pleasantly back into slumber.

We seem to be in perfect nighttime harmony. He nurses at night and I don't even wake up. Because of this, my life is so much easier than with my first baby.

Babies grow better. Sleep time is grow time for tiny babies. For over 150 years, pediatricians have noted that babies who sleep close to their mommies grow better. Here's some advice given in a childcare book written in 1840: "At least during the first four weeks . . . baby will thrive better if allowed to sleep beside its mother and cherished by her warmth than if placed in a separate bed." This was the "treatment" prescribed for "failure to thrive" babies. In my thirty years in pediatric practice, I have noticed that when cosleeping, a slow-gaining baby puts on more pounds. New insights into the fascinating interactions that go on between mother and baby when they share sleep shed light on the growth-promoting effects of cosleeping.

Babies get extra touch time when they share sleep with their mother. And "therapeutic touch" encourages growth. Also, babies who sleep close to their milk source naturally feed more frequently (smart babies!). And because Mom is more relaxed at night, she may deliver a higher-fat, and therefore higher-calorie, milk to baby. This high-fat milk is rich in brain-building omega-3 fats. (Remember, your milk-making hormones tend to be at higher levels during sleep.) When you sleep close to your baby and allow baby to nurse as needed, you deliver more "grow milk" and "smart milk" to your baby. The presence of their mother also stimulates the release of growth hormones in babies and lowers the levels of stress hormones, which interfere with growth.

Another reason why cosleepers grow better is that they waste less energy in nighttime restlessness. Studies by anthropologist James McKenna, director of the Mother-Baby Behavioral Sleep Laboratory at Notre Dame University, have exposed the myth that crib sleepers sleep more peacefully. Using videotapes of babies in different sleeping arrangements, Dr. McKenna showed that solo sleepers actually fret and squirm more than cosleepers. The last thing you want your preemie to do is waste energy squirming when he could be putting that energy into growing.

I coslept with him and became a sort of human apnea monitor. It made breastfeeding a lot easier and helped make up for all the time my son had to spend living in a plastic box.

Babies sleep more safely. Preemies, even when mature enough to leave the hospital, are prone to episodes of irregular breathing. Another name for this is periodic breathing. Babies may pause for ten to fifteen seconds between breaths and then breathe more rapidly for several breaths to catch up. They are also at risk for stop-breathing episodes, called apnea, when they may stop breathing for twenty seconds or more. The danger with apnea is that their breathing may not restart on its own. This is why premature babies with apnea are discharged with apnea monitors, which sound an alarm when baby pauses too long between breaths. Parents come running to pick baby up to restart his breathing. In rare instances, they even have to administer CPR. (Although apnea monitors haven't been proven to offer significant advantages to preemies and their parents, they are the only technology medicine has to offer to counteract apnea. Monitors often help parents and neonatologists worry less.)

My baby was born four weeks premature at 5 pounds 15 ounces. I held her and breastfed her all day long. She seemed perfectly healthy, pink, and breathed normally. That evening, when the pediatrician came to check her, she took her into the nursery and put her in the bassinet. As soon as our baby was lying in the bassinet alone, she had stop-breathing episodes, which alarmed the neonatologist, and she was put in intensive care for nine days. While in the NICU, all they had to do was touch her and she would start breathing again. She never had any stop-breathing episodes when she was in my arms, only when she was lying alone. When my baby was discharged, the doctors told me she was a prime candidate for SIDS. They convinced me that she needed to be on a home infant monitor. I agreed, but it turned out to be a nightmare for our whole family. I was told not to put her in my bed, so she slept alone with a monitor. The monitor went off all night long. After a while, I left her on the monitor but put her next to me and I slept with her side by side. We both slept wonderfully, and the monitor's alarm never sounded. I strongly feel that my presence stimulated her to breathe until she outgrew her stop-breathing tendencies. My touch and closeness to her was all she needed. In fact, while she was in my arms in the hospital all day long, no one ever knew she had a "breathing problem."

Having mother or father close by acting as a pacemaker is especially vital for preemies who are prone to irregular breathing and stop-breathing episodes. During the early months after birth, mother actually sleeps more lightly — "like a baby" — in order to compensate for the immaturity of baby's respiratory system. She fills in until baby is mature enough to sleep like an adult.

I (Dr. Bill) remember reading about an experiment many years ago that showed that infants with breathing difficulties, especially preemies, had fewer apnea episodes when placed next to a mechanically breathing teddy bear. I wondered, "Why not use the real human mother?"

My baby would breathe like a choo-choo train when sleeping alone. When I took him into our bed, he would breathe normally.

Dr. Bill's observations on cosleeping. Our fourth child, Hayden, was our first cosleeper. I became fascinated by observing what went on between her and her mother as they shared sleep. Martha would naturally put Hayden down to sleep on her back so that she could nurse more easily without completely waking up. Recent studies have shown that back-sleeping also lowers the risk of Sudden Infant Death Syndrome (SIDS), and public information campaigns about putting babies on their backs to sleep seem to be the prime explanation for a 50 percent reduction in the incidence of SIDS.

Sometimes Martha would sleep face-to-face with Hayden. I wondered if the face-to-face position could allow mother's breath to stimulate baby's breathing (more "magic breath"). I had noticed that when I breathed onto our babies' faces, they would take a deep breath. Researchers have recently discovered that the lining of baby's nose is rich in receptors that may affect breathing. Even more recent studies have shown that when mothers sleep face-to-face with their infants, the mother's breathing does stimulate baby's breathing.

Martha and Hayden seemed to be in sleep harmony, as if they were moving through the different stages of sleep together. I would see Hayden start to stir, and then Martha, prompted by some internal sensor, would turn toward Hayden, nurse or touch her, and the pair would drift back to sleep, often without completely awakening. Often I observed Hayden, still asleep but restless, reach out, touch Martha, take a deep breath, and resettle.

My observations of Martha and Hayden led me to believe that during sleepsharing, mother acts like a breathing pacemaker for her baby. By the time we had our eighth baby, and our fifth cosleeper, I was so fascinated by the mother-as-a-pacemaker theory that I decided to study it more scientifically. A local company provided technical assistance and the technology, and we set up equipment in our bedroom to monitor eight-week-old Lauren while she slept in two different arrangements. One night Martha and Lauren slept together in the same bed, as they usually did. The next night, Lauren slept in our bed and Martha slept in the adjacent room. Lauren's heart rate, breathing movements, the air flow from her nose, and her blood oxygen were monitored by a computer. This didn't appear to disturb her sleep. (We were able to monitor only Lauren's physiological changes during sleep, not Martha's.) A technician and I observed and recorded this physiological data. We then had it interpreted and analyzed by a pediatric pulmonary specialist who was blind to the study, which means he didn't know whether the data he was analyzing came from the solo-sleeping or shared-sleeping arrangement. Since this was the first time a cosleeping infant had been studied in the natural home environment as opposed to a sleep laboratory, I was invited to present these results at the International Apnea of Infancy conference in 1993.

Our study revealed that when Lauren was sleeping next to Martha, her breathing was more regular, her heart rate was more regular, there were fewer "dips" in her blood oxygen, and she had fewer stop-breathing, or slow-breathing episodes. The data from cosleeping were in striking contrast to the irregular respirations and frequent "dips" seen in the data gathered when Lauren was sleeping alone.

Dr. Jim says: I'm an avid sailor. People often ask me how a sailor gets any sleep when ocean-racing solo. While sleeping, the lone sailor puts the boat on autopilot. Because a sailor is so in tune with his boat, if the wind shifts so that something is not quite right with the boat, the sailor will automatically wake up. Perhaps the same safety awareness occurs between mother and her baby when they share sleep.

I automatically awaken just before my baby starts to stir, and I nurse her back to sleep. Usually neither of us fully awakens, and we both quickly drift back to sleep.

SCIENCE SAYS: SLEEP-SHARING IS BEST AND SAFEST FOR BABIES

Over the past decade, there have been more studies and interest in the physiological phenomenon of sleepsharing than ever before. Most of these studies have been performed by Dr. James McKenna, director of the Mother-Baby Behavioral Sleep Laboratory at Notre Dame University. Here's a summary of current sleepsharing research.

- Sleepsharing pairs tend to show more synchronous arousals than mother-and-baby pairs who sleep separately. This means when baby is about to awaken, mother also awakens. This synchrony allows mother to quickly resettle baby back to sleep, often without either member of the sleepsharing pair fully awakening.

- Mother and infant are often, but not always, in the same stage of sleep. When baby wakes up during the stage of light sleep, mother is also likely to be sleeping lightly. Mother resettles more easily than if she had been awakened from a deep sleep.

- Sleepsharing mothers do not get less total deep sleep than mothers who sleep separately.

- Babies tend to breastfeed more often when sleepsharing — a perk for preemies.

- Sleepsharing infants tend to spend more time sleeping on their backs or sides. These have been shown to be safer positions than on their tummies.

SAFE COSLEEPING WITH BABIES

If you choose to cosleep with your baby, observe these precautions:

- Place baby to sleep on her back (unless instructed otherwise by your baby's doctor).
- Enjoy a king-size bed. Use the money that you would have spent on a fancy crib and other less necessary baby furniture and treat yourself to a safe and comfortable king-size bed.
- While baby is unlikely to roll out of bed (like heat-seeking missiles, babies automatically gravitate toward a warm body), for safety's sake, place baby between mother and a mesh guardrail, or push the mattress flush against the wall. Be sure the guardrail is flush against the mattress, and be sure there are no crevices between the mattress and the headboard or wall.
- Tiny babies are usually safer placed between mother and the guardrail than between mother and father, since many fathers do not enjoy the keen awareness of baby's presence that mothers have.
- Don't fall asleep with baby on a couch, water bed, or any other cushiony surface.
- Don't sleep with your baby if you are under the influence of alcohol or medication that diminishes your awareness of baby.
- Never smoke where baby is sleeping.
- Don't allow a babysitter or older sibling to sleep with a tiny baby, as they don't enjoy the same natural keen awareness that mothers have.
- As an alternative to sleeping right next to your baby in bed, consider using an Arm's Reach Bedside Cosleeper, a bedside crib that attaches safely alongside your bed. This separate bed gives mother and baby their own sleeping space, yet keeps them within arm's reach for easy nursing and comforting. (See Bedside Cosleeper in Resources, page 235.)

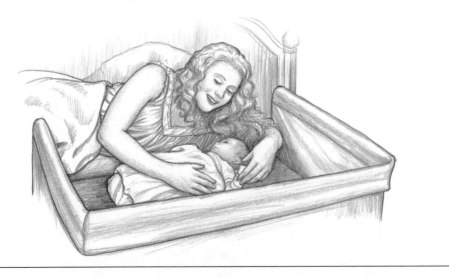

ALTERNATIVES TO CRIB SLEEPING

While nestled next to Mommy would likely be every baby's top choice, despite the benefits of sharing sleep with a preemie, not all parents are comfortable with that sleeping arrangement. Some worry that they will roll onto their baby or that their tiny baby will get lost in all the pillows and blankets. Most parents, however, are also reluctant to let their preemie sleep alone in another room. They want to be able to keep an eye on baby during the night. Besides the traditional options of a cradle, bassinet, or co-sleeper for having baby sleep nearby, consider this unique alternative:

Amby Baby Motion Bed. This new and creative option, developed in Australia and now available in the United States and many other countries, is a bassinet-size bed that hangs suspended by a spring and crossbar from a sturdy steel frame. We have already introduced you

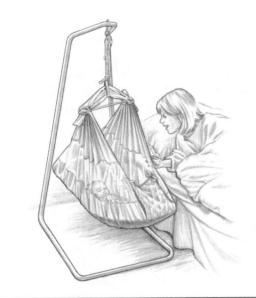

to how the Amby Bed can help your baby thrive while in the NICU (see page 74). Here are some continuing benefits you and your baby will enjoy if you choose this creative sleeping arrangement at home:

- Baby's slightly upright sleeping position minimizes the acid irritation that causes gastroesophageal reflux disease (GERD).
- Every time baby stirs or moves during sleep, the spring creates a gentle bouncing and rocking motion that lulls baby back to sleep.
- Gentle three-dimensional rocking motion imitates the womblike movement that baby craves.
- Instead of short, frequent naps, you and your baby can enjoy longer, uninterrupted naps each day.
- Baby feels more secure cuddled in the curve of the Amby Bed than in a large open and flat crib.
- Many preemies sleep better on their tummies, but this increases the risk of SIDS. The Amby Bed allows baby to sleep more comfortably on his back or side.
- The Amby Bed can be placed right next to your bed to give you access to baby during the night for feeding. You can easily bring baby into your bed as desired.

For more information, go to www. AmbyBaby.com.

6. Beware of Baby Trainers

As soon as you become parents, be prepared for a parade of well-meaning advisors, all showering you with their personal how-to's. Because you naturally want to give your premature baby the best parenting you can, you may be even more vulnerable to advice — some of which may help your parenting, some of which may hinder it. Beware especially of advice that puts distance — physical or emotional — between you and your baby. Parenting books and all kinds of advisors may promise that their methods will result in a baby who will "sleep through the night" and "feed on a predictable schedule." Their message is: "These babies will be less of a bother" and "You'll have more free time to yourself!" We call these advisors the "baby trainers." Baby training is similar to pet training, in both its methods and its goals. Baby training is not good for term babies, and it is particularly hazardous to the health of preemies. Here's why:

Baby training is biologically incorrect.
The first commandment of baby trainers is "Let your baby cry it out — don't rush to respond every time baby cries." Yet, as we have previously shown, crying it out is particularly harmful for preemies. Crying is physiologically stressful, and preemies don't need any more stress. Crying it out is not good for mothers either. It's easy for someone who has not shared an umbilical cord with your baby to tell you to ignore her cries. But a mother is biologically programmed to respond and not hold back when baby's cues say she is needed. When a baby cries, the blood flow to the mother's breasts increases, accompanied by a biological urge to pick up and comfort her baby. A mother who follows the baby-training regimen goes against her own biology, and she eventually desensitizes herself to her own instinctual knowledge of her baby. Insensitivity is just the opposite of what a mother of a preemie needs. Preemies have greater physiological needs than full-term babies, yet they are not as able to communicate these needs. A preemie needs her mother to build up her sensitivity, not tear it down.

"Scheduled feedings," another hallmark of baby training, are also biologically incorrect. Baby trainers have obviously never studied the physiology behind breastfeeding. The hormones that make milk have a short biological half life, which means they clear rapidly from mother's bloodstream. This suggests that babies are meant to breastfeed frequently and not on a strict schedule, to keep the hormone levels high. Feedings scheduled four hours apart may compromise baby's growth and mother's milk supply. Besides, tiny babies have tiny tummies, and premature intestines have immature digestive systems. So, more frequent and smaller feedings are just what preemies need.

Baby training keeps babies from thriving. Because all of their systems are immature and they have been born before their time, preemies go through a long period of catching up. To truly thrive, they must grow not only heavier and taller but also intellectually and emotionally. The low-touch style of baby training puts baby at risk for not thriving. A baby who does not receive the benefit of therapeutic touch and frequent feedings is at risk for not growing optimally. A baby whose cries are not listened to loses out on important lessons in early language. If no one responds to his signals, why try to communicate? Pediatricians even have a medical term for what can happen to a baby who is cut off from the closeness needed to grow optimally: failure to thrive. Over the years, I have noticed that some "trained" infants suffer from what I call "the shutdown syndrome." Here's one example:

Tom and Susan brought their three-month-old baby, Megan, into my office for a checkup. As they entered the exam room, I noticed they carried Megan in a plastic baby seat (clue #1) instead of their arms. As they sat next to my desk, they left Megan in her plastic seat a few feet away from them (clue #2). As they talked to me, there was little eye contact between Mother and Megan and Father and Megan (clue #3). Then Father exclaimed, "She sleeps through the night already" (clue #4), and Mother added, "And we've got her on a schedule" (clue #5). Finally, Dad said proudly, "And you know, Dr. Sears, she rarely cries" (clue #6). I was becoming concerned, but the parents seemed proud that they were raising such a "well-behaved" baby.

As I was examining Megan, I noticed she made very little eye contact with me, her muscle tone was not what I would have expected in a baby her age, and she had gained only 6 ounces over the past six weeks (the final clue). Megan was suffering from the shutdown syndrome. Because of long-distance parenting, Megan's physiological systems were operating at less than peak efficiency.

After listening to my talk on attachment parenting, Tom and Susan understood the simple value of touch and interaction. They had been led to believe that they were "disciplining" their baby with their parenting style and that this was good and necessary.

In looking back through Megan's chart, I noticed that these parents had started off with attachment parenting, and Megan had thrived in those early weeks. When they started imposing feeding and sleeping schedules and let her cry it out, she shut down. The parents had fallen into the wrong crowd of advisors and unknowingly pulled the plug on what was helping their baby thrive.

Within a month of returning to the Baby B's of attachment parenting, Tom and Susan had a thriving baby again.

7. Balance

In the zeal to give your baby "more," you will naturally have less time to meet your individual needs and those of your spouse. Each day, remind yourself that your baby needs two happy, rested parents. Remember, parents of premature babies are at higher risk for postpartum depression and burnout. Yet, in our pediatric practice we have found that more preemies who thrive have parents whose relationship is thriving also. Reserve enough time and energy to nurture yourself (whatever "just for me" activity you need) and your marriage (whatever "just for us" activity you need), and the final B of attachment parenting will help all the other six tools work better.

Both parents must also balance the time they spend caring for baby. Dads, when you come home from work, realize that Mom has been working all day. Take over the evening baby-wearing, diaper changing, feeding (if using bottles), and some of the night wakings. A burned-out mother will be less good for your baby and you.

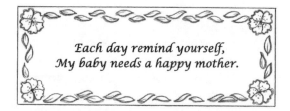

Each day remind yourself,
My baby needs a happy mother.

HOW ATTACHMENT PARENTING HELPS PREEMIES GROW — WHAT SCIENCE SAYS

The reason AP preemies grow better, breathe better, and do lots of other things better is because *attachment parenting organizes a preemie's physiology*. A preemie enters the world with immature physiological systems; the heart, lungs, central nervous system, endocrine system, digestive systems, and immune system operate at less than peak efficiency. The continued presence of an attachment person, usually a mother, though it can also be a father, lowers baby's stress level, so these systems function more efficiently. Mother's milk provides the nutrients needed for these systems to mature. Physical contact with Mother helps regulate body temperature and breathing and heart rates. Consider the term prematurity: born before the systems are mature. Parenting helps them mature. That's AP in a nutshell.

Over the past twenty years, I've had the opportunity to study attachment research, specifically research on the therapeutic benefits of the simple closeness of a mother to her prematurely born baby.

MORE!

During the journey of parenting your preemie, you will realize your baby needs more of everything — more feedings, more touch, more holding, more doctor visits, and more understanding and flexibility from you. In the early weeks at home, you may feel it's one big give-a-thon, and there will be days when you feel you may give out.

Yet, at some time in the first few weeks and months (maybe later), you will realize how much more your baby has given to you. In the process of parenting, you discover *mutual giving*. You give more — you get more. Because of the extra feedings and extra holding your baby requires, you become more sensitive to your preemie's needs and more aware of what makes her special. Parents of preemies call upon this heightened awareness all the time. They say "I feel . . ." or "I just know . . ." when describing what their baby is doing and why. In my early years as a pediatrician, I noticed during their frequent office visits that parents of preemies seemed to know their babies more intimately than many parents of term babies did. Challenged to become "monitors" of their babies' physiological changes, breathing patterns, heart rates, and less predictable feeding and sleeping schedules, these parents rose to the occasion. They taught me a valuable lesson about what I call the need-level concept. When a baby is born with a higher level of needs, parents — given appropriate information, tools, and support — will instinctively develop a higher level of parenting skills.

(Many of these studies were done on humans, and some on animals.) These fascinating studies often lie buried in scientific and medical journals and seldom make headlines in newspapers. Here are some of the highlights of what science says about a mother's role in adding the finishing touch to her preemie:

AP puts baby in better biochemical balance. Circulating throughout the bloodstream is an adrenal hormone called cortisol, which helps all the major organ systems of the body function optimally. These systems need the right amount of cortisol at the right times. Too much or too little and the body is not in tune, sort of like a car engine trying to run with the wrong mixture of fuel and air. Studies show that infants with the closest attachment to their mothers have the best cortisol balance. The longer infants are separated from their mothers, the higher their stress hormone levels. Prolonged elevations of cortisol may diminish growth and suppress the immune system.

AP stimulates growth hormones. Researchers learn a lot about the physiological benefits of mother-infant attachment by studying the effects of mother-infant separation. Infants separated from their mothers show physiological symptoms such as irregular heartbeats, irregular body temperature, and a decrease in REM sleep, the stage of sleep that stimulates brain growth. In studies of animals, infants who were closest to their mothers had the highest levels of growth hormones and enzymes essential for brain and heart growth. Separation from the mother or lack of interaction with the mother caused the levels of these growth-promoting biochemicals to fall. Even human infants deprived of sufficient interaction with an attachment figure may have lower levels of growth hormones. It follows then that attachment-parented babies are likely to have higher levels of growth-promoting hormones and the right balance of other hormones that help them thrive.

AP helps preemies conserve energy. In addition to having a better biochemical balance, an AP baby cries less and is less anxious, and therefore wastes less energy. The attached baby then has more energy for growing physically, physiologically, and intellectually. AP preemies don't just grow, they thrive.

AP helps baby's systems operate more efficiently. Attachment researchers use heart rate and variations in heart rate (how well the heart responds to changes in physiological needs) as indicators of a baby's physiological well-being. Attachment-parented newborns, especially breastfed babies, have been found to have lower heart rates, more efficient heart-rate variability, improved behavioral organization, and more organized and growth-promoting sleep than infants given a more detached style of parenting. Attachment researchers concluded that the Baby B's, especially breastfeeding and babywearing, help a newborn become more energy efficient. They compare the physiology of a less attached newborn to an automobile engine in need of a tune-up.

Common Concerns During the First Year

URING THE FIRST YEAR, preemies need all the care that term babies need and then some. Your preemie has a unique set of needs. In this chapter we will address common concerns about feeding, development, and caregiving shared by parents of preemies. You will learn a lot about your baby in this first year. Some of it will come from reading books and articles, some from talking with the various experts involved in your baby's care. But most of what you learn will come directly from your baby. The more time you spend with your baby, responding to her cues and watching her growth and development, the more confident you will feel as a parent and the more the two of you will enjoy each other.

FEEDING CONCERNS

Giving your preemie optimal nutrition is one of the most important things you can do to help her achieve optimal growth. As her tastes branch out from breast milk or formula to include other foods, you want to be sure that she continues to get the very best nutrition. Try these feeding tips:

Continue breastfeeding for at least one year. This isn't just our advice, it's the official recommendation of the American Academy of Pediatrics. During the first three years, baby's brain and nervous system grow more quickly than at any other time. The nutrients in breast milk not only promote brain growth but also foster the optimal growth of every other organ in your baby's body. Continue breastfeeding for as long as you and your baby are able. When baby starts solids, remember that these foods are an addition to, not a replacement for, the more valuable nutrition in breast milk. Many babies are happy to nurse past their second birthday and well into their third year of life. Extended breastfeeding provides toddlers with a nutritional and immunological boost, as well as the emotional reassurance they need as they grow. As long as you and your child are both happy with nursing, there is no reason to wean.

READ MORE!

Preemies have some unique needs, but first and foremost your preemie is a baby, like any other baby. And there's a lot more you will want to know about parenting your baby during the first two years. We suggest you consult *The Baby Book,* written by the Sears family: Dr. Bill and his wife, Martha, plus doctor sons Bob and Jim (Little, Brown, revised and updated 2003). In this 770-page reference book, you will find detailed information about many of the parenting topics covered in this book, as well as additional information about caring for babies and toddlers. Topics include:

- how to get your baby to sleep
- parenting the fussy or colicky baby
- enjoying and maximizing your baby's developmental stages
- general medical care
- tips for becoming your family's nutritionist
- CPR — a step-by-step illustrated guide

Read, read, read! While some people advise against it for fear that you may get scared by all the things that can go wrong, because I was informed, I didn't get as upset as my husband, who didn't read as much.

Give baby enough formula. If baby is formula-fed, formula will remain an important part of his diet until he is one year of age. After you have figured out which formula and feeding techniques work best for you and your baby, gradually increase the amount of formula your baby takes. Even after he is 6 months of age, try to give your baby a minimum of 32 ounces of formula each day until he is one year of age.

As baby's appetite increases, do not be tempted to decrease the amount of formula and increase the amount of solid foods. Consider solid foods to be an addition to baby's diet, not a substitute for formula. Solid foods cannot provide all the nutrients that are in formula.

Always give your baby an iron-fortified and DHA/ARA-enriched formula, and avoid changing formulas, unless advised to do so by baby's health care provider. If you are using a special formula for preemies, your baby may or may not need extra iron and vitamins. Be sure to check with your doctor. Wait until baby is at least one year of age before switching to whole cow's milk.

Give baby enough iron. Because they were born before they could store enough iron, preterm babies usually need iron supplements, given daily in the form of drops, for at least the first 6 months. During baby's routine office visits, your doctor will check her hemoglobin and adjust the iron dosage accordingly. Both breastfeeding and formula-feeding preemies need iron supplements until at least 6 months of age. When you begin giving your baby solid foods, include those with high levels of iron: prune juice, iron-fortified cereals, tofu, sweet potatoes, and puréed beef and chicken.

Give your baby extra vitamins and minerals. Most preemies are given a liquid multivitamin and -mineral preparation when they go home from the NICU. This supplementation is necessary to make up for the nourishment in the womb that baby missed out on because of his premature birth. The extra vitamins and minerals are also needed for catch-up growth in the first year. We suggest you continue giving your baby a vitamin and mineral supplement for at least the first year or two.

Delay solids until at least 6 months of age. The American Academy of Pediatrics recommends that infants not start solids until after their 6-month birthday. This applies to preemies as well as full-term infants. We suggest you wait to offer solids until your baby is 6 months' *gestational age.* For example, if your baby was born 2 months early, wait until baby is 8 months old to offer solid food. Why wait? There are several reasons. First, breast milk and formula contain more nutrients than solid foods, so they should be baby's main source of nutrition in the first year. Second, research has shown that infants whose intestines are exposed to anything besides breast milk or formula before 6 months of age are more likely to develop allergies later in childhood. Third, giving baby too much solid food too soon can lead to constipation, which is not only uncomfortable for baby but can cause bloating that is

EXTRA FAT FOR EXTRA GROWTH

If your baby needs extra calories for growth, provide them in the form of extra fat. Each gram of fat contains 9 calories, compared with 4 calories per gram of protein and carbohydrates. In our pediatric practice, we frequently suggest that parents of a baby who needs to grow add from 1 to 3 teaspoons of flaxseed oil to baby's daily diet. This can be mixed into baby's formula or, for babies 6 months and older, stirred into solid food. Flaxseed oil contains valuable nutrients, such as omega-3 fats, in addition to extra calories. Teach baby's young taste buds to appreciate it. Later on, you can add a tablespoon of flaxseed oil to a fruit-and-yogurt smoothie to get more calories into a picky eater.

"But shouldn't my baby be on a low-fat diet?" you might be wondering. "Isn't everyone supposed to be on a low-fat diet?" No, not everyone. The low-fat label has no place in feeding infants, especially not in feeding preemies. Fifty percent of the calories in breast milk come from fat, and when it comes to nutrition, nature makes no mistakes. Babies need fat to grow and to build strong body tissues. Instead of a low-fat diet for your infant, think right-fat diet. Best fats for babies, especially preemies, are:

- human milk — the gold standard!
- flaxseed oil
- salmon, wild
- oils from plant sources, such as olive oil and vegetable oils (nonhydrogenated)
- avocados

severe enough to compromise breathing. If your thriving infant seems eager to get at what's on your plate at 4 or 5 months of age, give him a spoon or cup to play with. Wait a few more months before you share your mashed potatoes.

Offer "grow foods." When it's time for baby to try new foods, follow the "more for less" feeding principle. Because tiny babies have tiny tummies (about the size of their fist), offer nutrient-dense foods: those that pack a lot of nutrition into small servings. In the chart below are some examples and when to start feeding them.

Shape tiny taste buds. As much as possible, make your own baby food. The first two years are a window of opportunity for shaping your child's tastes. If your infant's developing taste buds are exposed only to nutritious homemade food during these formative years, your baby will regard homemade food as the norm (this is what real food is supposed to taste like!). Your child is then more likely to grow up preferring the taste of whole foods rather than processed ones. An infant whose diet is composed primarily of canned, jarred, and processed foods accepts these artificial tastes as the norm and may shun the more nutritious "grow foods" that Mom makes. Instead of starting baby on bland rice cereal or processed baby food, let him try some interesting fresh foods, such as soft steamed carrots, mashed sweet potatoes, or mashed bananas. These are colorful and full of intriguing flavors. A baby who is exposed to a variety of flavors (rather than bland processed baby food that all tastes the same) is more likely to become an adventurous eater.

Don't force-feed. Some preemies have an oral aversion; they are sensitive about what goes into their mouth and may reject

6 to 9 months*	9 to 12 months*	12 months*
• applesauce • avocados • bananas • barley cereal • carrots • flaxseed oil • oatmeal • papaya • pears • prunes • rice cereal • squash • sweet potatoes	• brown rice • chicken (puréed) • egg yolk (omega-3 enriched) • lamb • pasta • peas • tofu • turkey • yogurt (without corn syrup or artificial sweeteners)	• beef (puréed) • broccoli • cheese • cottage cheese • eggs, whole • mango • melon • salmon, wild • spinach • tomatoes • whole-grain bread
* Gestational, not chronological, age		

anything that isn't a nipple. Part of this is due to immaturity, and part may be a reaction to unpleasant experiences in the NICU. If your baby does not seem interested in solids or rejects them completely, don't push it. Nothing makes a picky eater more picky than being forced to eat. You may also find that your baby doesn't like foods with certain consistencies and isn't progressing through the baby food "stages" as the baby food advertisers say he should. Don't worry if your preemie prefers nothing but puréed foods until one year of age, or even beyond. Eventually he will be willing to try other textures. Your doctor or occupational therapist can give you some tips on introducing new foods to your reluctant eater.

DEVELOPMENTAL CONCERNS

"Will my preemie develop differently from a full-term baby?" is a common concern we hear from parents. Yes, your baby will progress at his own rate and in his own style through the usual developmental milestones. Remember that even in term babies, there is a wide range of norms for which skills develop when. When you consider your preemie's developmental progress, keep the following factors in mind:

READ MORE!

There's lots more to learn about good nutrition for growing children. For a crash course on how to become your family's own nutritionist, read *The Family Nutrition Book,* by William Sears and Martha Sears (Little, Brown, 1999).

Your baby's gestational age. Look at ages for attaining developmental milestones in terms of your baby's gestational age, not his chronological age, just as your baby's pediatrician does in plotting your baby's growth on a standardized growth chart. For example, most term babies are able to sit unsupported at around 6 months of age. If your baby was born 2 months early, he may not sit up by himself until 8 months.

Your baby's own progress. Progress is more important than developmental "deadlines." Instead of focusing on when your baby does what, enjoy the fact that each month she is doing more than she was the previous month. While her progress may be a month or two behind that of a full-term baby, she will follow the same sequence of development. As you watch your baby grow, you will notice that she can do more and more as the weeks go by. You'll see more eye contact, more interest in playing with you and following your movements, and more hand play. When playing on the floor, she will gradually be able to get more and more of her body off the ground. Her new sounds and facial gestures will delight you and make her more fun to be with as the months go by.

Make your own chart. As a guideline in creating your chart, use the headings on the developmental chart on page 172, which was designed for full-term babies. Down the left side of your page, list the areas of development (i.e., gross motor, fine motor, social and language). Across the top, label the columns by baby's age in months. Then, as the months go by, jot down notes about your baby's accomplishments in each area of development.

When you compare this month with last month, you will notice that baby is making progress. Some months you will see more progress in the area of fine motor skills; other months the big news will be social, language, or gross motor development. When you compare your baby's chart with the standard chart for full-term infants, be sure to correct for baby's gestational age. The accomplishments you list on your chart at 8 months of age will probably be similar to those listed for full-term babies who are 6 months old. Eventually, the gap between your baby and full-term infants with the same chronological age will narrow.

Preemies are at a higher risk of developmental delay than their full-term peers are. While the reasons for this are not entirely clear, it seems that some nerves in the brains of preemies do not form all the necessary connections as quickly as they would if baby had been born full-term. Your pediatrician will track your baby's development closely. Most preemies will also have a scheduled evaluation with a team of doctors, nurses, and developmental therapists in the NICU "follow-up clinic" one or more times during the first year of life. Or, your baby's development may be monitored by therapists and other specialists in an Early Intervention Program (see page 174). Any concerns you may have about your baby's development can be evaluated and addressed by these professionals.

Dr. Bob advises: Forget the "should be doing's" for each month and enjoy what your baby *is* doing. Make a chart or keep a diary about your baby's development. Take your personal preemie chart with you to scheduled visits with your doctor, therapist, or Early Intervention Program. Your observations about your baby's development are just as important as, or even more important than, the observations of specialists who see your baby for only a short period of time. Some of the assessment tools used by developmental specialists depend heavily on interviews with baby's caregiver. You may be asked, "Can baby do this? Can baby do that? And when did he start doing this or that?" You'll find it easier to answer these questions accurately if you can refer to your notes. Also, if your baby is sleepy or fussy during an evaluation, the therapist or doctor will not get a true picture of baby's abilities, and your report becomes even more important. Development is most accurately assessed when a baby is in a state of quiet alertness. This is why it's best to schedule visits with your doctors and others for the morning — or whatever time of day your experience tells you your baby will be at his best.

Don't worry about developmental milestones in the first year. Just enjoy your baby!

Promoting preemie development through parenting. If your baby already has some delays in development or is at high risk of having developmental challenges, your interactive, sensitive attachment parenting is more important than ever. Physical, occupational, and speech therapists, plus medical specialists, will be involved in your baby's care, but through all of this, who is going to be spending the most time with baby? Who is going to be the single most influential source of stimulation for baby? You, the parent. You have been at the center of your baby's Early Intervention Program since the first time

	1 month	2 months	4 months	6 months	9 months	12 months
Gross motor	Lifts head slightly	Lifts head more	Lifts head to 90 degrees and scans environment Stands supported	Sits briefly by self Needs help to stand yet supports most of weight on legs	Crawls Pulls self up to stand	Cruises, holding on to furniture Takes a few steps Walks assisted
Fine motor	Hands remain in tight fists	Visually tracks parents Unfolds hands Briefly grasps toys	Embraces and reaches with both hands Holds toys longer Brings toys toward mouth	Transfers toys from one hand to the other Has more accurate reach and grab	Picks up objects with thumb and forefinger Points to toys	Feeds self, holding bottle or cup to drink
Social and language	Smiles occasionally Startles, turns toward sounds	Coos, squeals Holds eye contact, studies faces	Laughs Enjoys social gesturing (e.g., flapping arms to be picked up) Tracks moving objects Engages in more eye contact	Imitates facial gestures Looks at mirror image Begins babbling	Waves bye-bye Babbles more, may begin to say words (e.g., "ma-ma," "da-da")	May say a few intelligible words (e.g., "ba" for ball) Points and gestures for help Recognizes and points to familiar persons at the sound of their names

you held your preemie in the hospital. The developmental and emotional stimulation that you provide day in and day out will mean more to baby's success than all the input from professionals put together.

NINE WAYS TO HELP YOUR PREEMIE'S DEVELOPMENT

Your own individual parenting ideas and skills, along with the tools of attachment parenting presented in chapter 10, will help you build a brighter, healthier, happier baby. Here are nine ways parents and other caregivers can promote baby's development:

1. Provide smarter milk. As we discussed in detail in chapter 6, mother's milk is rich in brain-building fats, dubbed smart fats. Since research has shown that the more frequently and the longer infants are breastfed, the healthier and smarter they are, breastfeed your baby as frequently and as long as you can. If you are combining breastfeeding and formula-feeding or are exclusively formula-feeding, use a DHA/ARA-enriched infant formula.

2. Provide smarter food. A baby's brain triples in size during the first year and then doubles in size again by five years of age. How you feed the brain during these early years affects the quality of its growth.

When your baby is ready for solid foods (after 6 months of age), concentrate on smart nutrition:

- *Feed your baby smart fats.* Beginning around one year, feed your baby a couple ounces of wild Alaskan salmon two or three times a week. Not only is salmon from the pristine waters of Alaska rich in brain-building omega-3 fats, it's likely to be mercury- and pesticide free.
- *Start your baby's day off with a brainy breakfast.* Studies show that children pay better attention and learn complex tasks more easily when they begin the day with a smart nutritional start. A smart breakfast includes a balance of proteins, complex carbohydrates, and healthy fats. Some brainy breakfasts are: Eggs, whole wheat toast, and fruit; and cereal, yogurt, and fruit.
- *Shun junk foods.* One of the keys to optimal development is having stable blood sugar and insulin levels, and keeping the arteries to all the vital organs free of fats that can clog them. Beware of what we call the "terrible two's" of junk food: (1) foods and beverages sweetened with sugar and high-fructose corn syrup; and (2) foods containing hydrogenated fats and oils. Foods containing these ingredients generally have no place in childhood nutrition, especially not in the diet of preemies. Get used to shopping only the perimeter of the supermarket, where all the "grow foods" tend to be: fruits and veggies, seafood, eggs, and dairy products.

3. Wear your baby smartly in a carrier. Babies learn a lot while worn by a busy caregiver. Wear your baby in a sling wherever you go, and instruct other caregivers to do likewise. Babywearing fosters the state of quiet alertness, the behavioral state in which babies interact and learn best from their environment (see page 152).

4. Talk smart to your baby. Interactions, especially verbal, with other human beings, require the growing brain to make connections. The more connections that are made and the more they hook up into circuits, the smarter the brain becomes. It's as simple as that. Talk with your baby. During your daily activities, tell baby about what you're doing: "Now Daddy is putting a new diaper on baby"; "Let's put these pretty flowers on the table." During conversation, engage your baby in eye-to-eye contact. Sing to her. Exaggerate your body language and facial gestures. Remember, every piece of information babies take in requires them to make new connections. Do everything you can to be sure your baby lives in an information-rich environment.

5. Read to your baby. The more senses that are involved in interaction, the more brain connections your baby is required to make. When you look at books together, baby takes in more than just the words and pictures on the page. She also enjoys the sound of your voice and the closeness of sitting on your lap. Interactive activity books are great, too. Wrap these up in the joy you two share when you are together and you have a high-quality learning activity.

6. Play smart. Your baby's formal Early Intervention Program (see next page) may include infant stimulation classes — play sessions appropriate to her developmental level. At home, don't think of play as therapy. Make it fun.

7. Play with smart toys. Toys are an important part of the information-rich environment you are creating for your baby. Interesting interactions with toys build more pathways in the brain. Encourage your baby to have fun with toys that are based on the principle of cause and effect: "When I do something, something else happens." Simple blocks and balls are the best toys for older babies and toddlers. Everything they do depends on what baby does with them. They are also great toys for two: toys that parent and baby can enjoy together. See the Bright Starts section at www.AskDrSears.com for more development-enhancing play tips.

8. Play music. Music has an organizing effect on brain function. Babies prefer soothing classical music, especially Mozart and Bach. They also love songs sung by Mom and Dad. Take a simple nursery tune and make up your own repetitive sing-song words. Your baby will love it.

9. Get smart help. The Early Intervention Program in your community is a very helpful resource for parents of preemies. The Early Intervention staff can help you — your baby's first and most important teacher — do your job more effectively.

EARLY INTERVENTION PROGRAMS

The Early Intervention Program (EIP) is a federal- and state-funded program for infants who are at risk for developmental delay. The staff consists of social workers, occupational and physical therapists, speech pathologists, nutritionists, nurses, and doctors who will guide you and your baby through the first three years of life.

These experts will monitor your baby's developmental progress, educate you on ways to stimulate baby's development, provide services to those infants who are delayed, and identify babies who may need more extensive medical evaluation. At age three, your child will graduate from the EIP into early childhood education services provided by the public school system for preschoolers with developmental delays.

Here are some questions you may have about EIPs:

Which babies are eligible for an EIP?

Infants who are known to have developmental delays and infants who are at risk of developmental delays qualify for help from Early Intervention Programs. A preemie may fall into either one of these two categories. Those born extremely premature and those who have certain medical challenges qualify for EIP. Babies who show developmental delay as they grow also receive assistance.

What about premature babies who are discharged from the NICU healthy and thriving without any developmental or medical challenges?

These babies may not initially qualify for an Early Intervention Program. They are, however, at risk for developmental delay and would benefit from receiving services to prevent delays. Unfortunately, there may not be enough federal funding to include these babies in EIPs. The degree of federal funding varies from state to state, and it's up to state governments to decide whether or not to provide *preventive* EIP services to healthy premature babies.

How do I enroll my baby in an EIP?

One of the best ways to get your baby into an Early Intervention Program is to ask the NICU social worker to arrange for your baby to be evaluated by your local EIP center. The social worker can make the call for you, or you can call yourself to arrange an appointment. Do this while your baby is still in the NICU. If your baby does have certain medical problems that automatically qualify her for services, the medical staff can communicate directly with the EIP case worker or provide records of your baby's condition. If your baby does not have any medical conditions that automatically qualify her for EIP, the NICU social worker may still be able to get you an appointment for an evaluation. If you don't arrange for Early Intervention services at discharge from the NICU, your pediatrician can refer you to an Early Intervention Program if your baby begins to show signs of developmental delay.

How does an EIP work?

Programs vary from state to state, and even within a state. The services that are available depend greatly on the amount of state funding. Here are some general features of EIPs that will give you an idea of what to expect:

• *Caseworkers.* In most programs, your caseworker is your main contact. This person may be a social worker or a child development specialist. He or she will arrange for the initial evaluation, talk with you about your family situation and your baby's needs, and help determine what services your child will re-

ceive. He or she will also monitor your child's progress over time and arrange regular meetings between you and the staff.

• *Physical and occupational therapy.* Children with motor-skill delays and other medical conditions will receive physical therapy (PT) and/or occupational therapy (OT) to help them achieve optimal development. Your child may see the therapist as often as several times a week or only once or twice each month, depending on his needs. Some programs will send a therapist to your home, and some will provide services at a state-funded center or with a private therapist. The physical or occupational therapist will work directly with your child to improve his muscle strength, coordination, and developmental skills, and also teach you how to do these exercises with your baby in between therapy sessions.

• *Speech pathology.* A speech pathologist may work with you and your child on developing early language skills. Again, services may be provided in your home or at an EIP facility.

• *Regional therapy centers.* In some states, Early Intervention Programs are centralized, with large facilities for providing services and hundreds of caseworkers, therapists, nurses, and doctors involved. In less populated areas, there may not be a specific EIP center. Instead, a caseworker will help you find the needed services in your community.

• *Preschools.* Some programs will enroll your child in a special preschool staffed by educators and therapists who are specially trained in child development.

• *Group therapy.* Some programs will encourage you to participate with other parents and children in regularly scheduled group sessions led by various developmental specialists.

• *Home visits.* In some situations, caseworkers will make scheduled home visits to assess your child's progress. They may even arrange for your child to receive certain aspects of therapy in your home, depending on your child's needs.

How important is an EIP?

Research has shown that at-risk or developmentally delayed infants who receive EIP services attain developmental milestones faster or score higher on developmental tests (particularly in intellectual development) during the first few years of life. What is not yet known is whether these early gains make a significant long-term difference. Studies that compare children who were enrolled in an EIP as infants with those who were not enrolled show very little difference between the two groups in IQ and behavioral problems later in childhood. Still, it stands to reason that years of speech, physical, occupational, and developmental therapy services can help a developmentally delayed or at-risk child, and they certainly can't hurt. Most parents and medical professionals agree that EIP services are extremely valuable, even though there is not yet any solid research to confirm this belief. Hopefully, ongoing research will validate the importance of Early Intervention Programs for our nation's children and demonstrate their cost effectiveness.

TRAVELING WITH PREEMIES — WHEN AND HOW?

Once you finally arrive home with your baby, the last thing you may want to do is leave home. Yet, travel is an inevitable part of modern life, so you need to be prepared.

Car Travel

You and your baby are likely to spend a significant amount of time in the car, traveling to appointments with various health care providers. Be sure to restrain your baby in a car seat or car bed whenever she is in the car. Most car seats are designed for larger babies, so not all of the infant seats on the market will work well with preemies. Preemies have weaker head and neck control than full-term babies, so their heads flop forward and sideways during the stops and swerves of normal driving. The bent and slumped position that preemies end up in while riding in a car seat can compromise their breathing and aggravate reflux. Here's how to work around these car seat quirks:

Try before you buy. Many NICUs have one or more car seats that you can "try on" your preemie while still in the hospital.

Test before you buy. Many NICUs monitor baby's oxygen saturation and heart rate in the car seat a day or two before anticipated discharge, especially if baby is prone to apnea, bradycardia, and/or reflux. While they are monitoring baby in the car seat, it's possible to experiment with different positions, from semi-reclining (45 degrees) to fully reclining, as in a car bed. Trying and testing car seats and car beds allows you to select the optimal reclining angle for safest travel. If baby is too close to horizontal in a conventional car seat, there will not be enough back support to restrain baby in the case of a head-on collision.

WEIGHING ADVICE FROM THE EXPERTS

The professionals who work with you and your baby in your Early Intervention Program know a great deal about how to encourage babies to learn new skills. They are experts on baby's development of motor skills, speech and language, and thinking. But you are the expert on your baby and on the kind of parenting your baby needs. If advice from your baby's therapists goes against your parenting instincts, think long and hard about what is best for your baby. For example, the physical therapist may suggest that you not carry your baby all the time, so that she has opportunities to move her body in many directions. You may feel that your baby is most comfortable in the baby sling and that she really does not want to be put down. How do you resolve this conflict?

It may be helpful to talk with the therapist about the reasons for giving baby "floor time." You can also explain how much stimulation your baby gets while she is in the sling. Perhaps you and the therapist can work together on finding ways your baby can be encouraged to use her muscles to support more of her body while in the sling. Similarly, the speech pathologist may want to encourage baby to try new tastes and textures in food, while you want to encourage baby to breastfeed for as long as possible. Again, use your own best judgment to weigh the advice, find out more about the reasons behind it, and work together with the therapist to come up with a plan that suits your baby and your parenting values.

On the other hand, if baby is too close to vertical, her head could flop forward, especially if the car comes to a sudden stop. For many preemies, the optimal reclining angle for a car seat is around 45 degrees. (To achieve this angle, you may have to wedge a firm towel roll underneath the front of the car seat.) Preemies with unstable breathing may need to be placed in a fully reclining car bed rather than a car seat, at least for the first month or two.

Car seat or car bed? Preemies who do better in a car bed are those who have:

- unstable breathing (apnea, bradycardia) when in a car seat
- low or "floppy" muscle tone
- a cast or brace

We used suction-cup rearview mirrors to help keep a watchful eye on our rear-facing baby in the backseat.

Properly position your preemie. After you've selected the optimal reclining angle, add padding around baby's head and sides to center baby in the car seat, as shown in the illustration.

Be sure that distance between the crotch strap and the back of the car seat is no more than 5½ inches, and that the distance from the bottom of the harness strap to the floor of the car seat is no more than 10 inches. Otherwise, the straps could come alongside baby's ears instead of being at shoulder height. Put the shoulder straps in the lowest slots until your baby grows taller. Place the retainer clip at the midpoint of baby's chest, not too close to the neck area or too low on the abdomen.

Pad your preemie. Besides putting padding alongside baby's head, using folding diapers, towels, blankets, or commercially available inserts, pad the car seat's harness straps. (Commercial harness pads are available at infant product stores and web sites.) If there's still a lot of slack between baby's diaper area and the crotch strap, wedge in a folded cloth diaper to keep her from slipping down. Do not add padding under or behind the infant to make the seat fit the baby.

Position baby in the car safely. The safest place is the middle of the backseat. Never place a car seat in the front seat when there is a passenger-side air bag.

Buckle up. Use only car seats with a 3-point or 5-point harness system. Do not

use a safety seat with a shield or abdominal pad. In the case of a sudden stop or a collision, a preemie's head could flop against the shield, causing injury.

Wire up. If your baby is being sent home with an apnea monitor, be sure it is portable and that you understand how to use it while baby is positioned in the car seat. Also, find out how long the battery power will last and make sure it is fully charged before long car trips.

Keep an eye on your baby. Because of potential breathing problems in the slumped position in the car seat, never leave a baby unattended in a car seat. When you must drive alone with baby, place a suction mirror on the rear window so you can observe baby when you stop in traffic.

Follow instructions. Be sure to get a government-approved car seat and follow

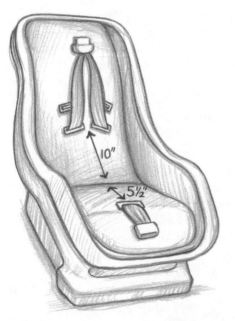

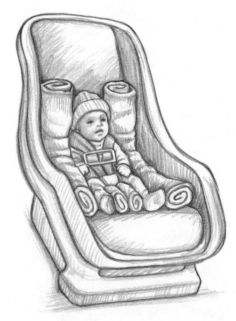

the manufacturer's instructions. Because of frequent changes in styles of infant safety car seats, as well as periodic recalls, we have chosen not to mention brands. Choose a car seat recommended by the NICU staff or check for periodic updates at www.AskDrSears.com/preemies.

Air Travel

It's generally wise to put off air travel until your preemie is at least 9 months of age, depending on baby's overall medical condition and the advice of your baby's doctor. The air in the cabin of an airplane usually has a slightly lower oxygen level than outside air. While this may not be a problem for many babies, it may not be good for preemies whose oxygen saturations are already marginal. Also, avoid traveling to high-altitude locations, where the oxygen saturation in the air is less than baby is accustomed to.

Infection control is another important air travel issue. Most airplanes now recycle cabin air, which is more economical than processing outside air. Recycled cabin air may contain more germs. Also, the notoriously low humidity of cabin air can dry and clog baby's breathing passages.

Here are some tips for when you must travel by air with your baby:

- Ask to be seated next to an empty seat if possible. If the plane is not full, the agent will usually oblige.
- While the plane is moving on the ground, keep baby in a car seat if the seat is open next to you. This will keep her safe if the plane comes to a sudden stop.
- Since sucking and swallowing can lessen ear pain, feed baby during take-off and

landing, especially during landing, as a change in air pressure can plug the eustachian tubes and cause ear pain. If she is sleeping, let her stay asleep. Waking a sleeping baby is likely to cause her to cry more than the possible discomfort in her ears will.

- Tank up baby with a full feeding before you board the plane. During the flight, offer smaller, more frequent feedings to minimize overswallowing of air. Lower cabin pressure at high altitudes can cause the air in the intestines to expand, causing bloating and colicky abdominal pain.
- Keep baby's breathing passages moist by placing a warm, moist washcloth near her nose and spritz a couple of drops of saltwater nose drops (available at your pharmacy as "nasal saline drops") into each of her nostrils at least every hour.
- Wear baby in a sling to discourage curious passersby from touching her. When standing in a crowded line, cover her with the sling to minimize exposure to germs in the air.

PARENTING TWINS AND MULTIPLES

Twins, triplets, and multiples are likely to be born early, so many parents of preemies bring more than one baby home from the NICU. As the number of babies goes up, so do the challenges. Your first year as parents of multiples will be exhausting, and your memories of these months will be a bit of a blur. Here are some tips to survive and thrive as the parents of more than one baby.

Dad doubles as "Mom." With multiples, Dad has no choice but to be heavily involved in baby care. The only mothering task that Dad can't do is breastfeed. Everything else can, and must, be shared by both parents if the whole family is going to grow and thrive.

Be doubly prepared. Double the diapers, double the laundry, double the feedings. Two or more babies mean that you need more of everything. As discharge day approaches, make sure you have everything you are going to need at home for your babies. There won't be time for quick shopping trips once your multiples are at home.

Don't forget that your babies' at-home caregivers (that's you, Mom and Dad!) also need to be cared for. While you're stocking up on diapers and baby equipment, stock up on things that will keep you well fed and happy. Collect take-out menus from your favorite restaurants. Stock your freezer and pantry with healthy snacks and the ingredients for quick, easy meals. Find a supermarket or online service that will deliver groceries to your door. Buy some good-looking, easy-care clothing that you can pull on in the morning without thinking. (Prints will camouflage leaking milk and spit-up.) Anything that makes life easier for you will make life better for your babies, since what they need most are relaxed and happy parents.

Be doubly organized. The stress of caring for one baby can turn a mother's mind to mush, at least temporarily. Multiples make mothers' minds even mushier. Don't worry, your brain will eventually learn to cope with the complexity of parenting twins or triplets. But in the meantime, you may want to keep daily charts of who was

fed and changed when, who spit up or seemed in pain, and anything else that you may want to discuss with the babies' pediatrician or other caregivers.

Get help. When friends or family members offer to help, don't turn them down. Be ready with suggestions. Keep a list near the phone of errands or household jobs that others can do for you. Perhaps one friend or family member could be in charge of organizing a schedule for others to bring you meals, run errands, or entertain older siblings. Hire household help. For parents of multiples, this is not a luxury, it's a necessity. If looking at dust bunnies and fingerprints on kitchen cabinets makes you depressed, pay someone to do it for you.

Take advantage of backup arms. Preemie twins and triplets like to be held as much as singletons do. Invest in two baby slings, one for Mom and one for Dad. Then the two of you can wear your babies in slings when you need to get out of the house. Wearing your babies around the house is a good way to keep them content. If one wakes up from a nap crying, quickly pop him into the sling before his cries awaken his brother or sister. If you need to hold two babies at once, put one in the sling and hold the other in your free arm. Until your babies are ready to get around on their own, you will seldom be without a baby riding on your hip or draped over your shoulder.

Fortunately, moms and dads are not the only adults who enjoy holding babies. While you don't want to pass your preemies off to anyone and everyone who wants to hold them for a few minutes, you will appreciate the willing arms of a few good baby soothers. Line up some baby-holding help from grandparents and others, especially in the late afternoon, when babies are likely to be fussy and moms and dads are tired.

If anyone asks, "Do you need anything?" say, "Yes, can you please come over and hold one of the babies?"

Get some support. Your local Mothers of Twins Club is a good source of both emotional support and practical advice. You'll meet other moms of multiples at the meetings, many of whom will have experience with parenting preemies. (See Twins and Multiples in Resources, page 236.)

Establish sleep routines. You can't force babies to fall asleep at the same time, but you can set the stage for this to happen. Establish two or three times during the day when all of you will lie down together. Play the same soft, soothing music you shared with your babies in the NICU, nurse them, stroke their backs, and rest and relax yourself. You need this time to wind down as much as the babies do.

Consider co-bedding. Once your babies are stable and in the grower nursery, try placing them side by side or face-to-face in the same bassinet. Continue this sleep-sharing arrangement at home. After all, they were "womb mates" for seven or eight months. Co-bedding stabilizes their breathing and heart rates and regulates their temperatures. A 2002 study showed that preterm twins had fewer apnea episodes when co-sleeping. Many neonatologists feel that co-bedding multiples grow faster and seem happier than those

who sleep separately. Co-bedding may also help your babies get on similar sleep schedules.

Breastfeeding More Than One Preemie

Will you be able to breastfeed your preemie twins (or triplets or more)? Your body can make enough milk for two, and many mothers of full-term breastfed twins do manage to exclusively breastfeed for many months. How well breastfeeding works for your preemies will depend on a number of factors: how premature your babies are, how eagerly they take to the breast, how successful you are at keeping up your milk supply by pumping, and how much time it takes to feed your babies.

Even if you can produce only half the milk they need, congratulate yourself on that half rather than worrying about the half you can't produce.

For many mothers of preemies, the hardest part of breastfeeding is the transition from pumping and gavage feeding to feeding baby at the breast. Teaching even one baby to latch on and suck effectively can be very time-consuming. At each feeding, you have to work with baby and get her to latch on and suck, then feed baby the required supplement, then pump your breasts to keep up your milk supply. By the time you store the pumped milk and clean the pump parts, it's almost time to do it all again. With two or more babies, this routine may be more than one mother can handle, and it may be necessary to find a way to combine breastfeeding with bottlefeeding. Here are some suggestions for simplifying feedings when there's more than one mouth to feed:

- Dad can give one baby a bottle while Mom breastfeeds the other. At the next feeding, switch babies.
- As your babies get older and more proficient at nursing, you may be able to breastfeed both at the same time. A breastfeeding pillow that fits around your middle will help you support both babies at your breasts. See *The Breastfeeding Book,* by William Sears and Martha Sears (Little, Brown, 2000), for instructions and illustrations of positions for breastfeeding two babies at once.
- One baby may be more successful at learning to breastfeed than the other. That baby may get her milk directly from the breast while her sibling gets formula or expressed breast milk in a bottle.
- Rigid feeding schedules usually aren't good for babies, but cue-feeding two may be too chaotic for parents. Try to find a balance. If one baby is hungry and wants to be fed, offer a feeding to the other as well. You'll buy some time this way.
- Get expert help, right from the start. The hospital's lactation consultant can help and support you through the challenges of breastfeeding more than one baby. La Leche League International's book *Mothering Multiples: Breastfeeding and Caring for Twins or More,* by Karen Gromada, contains detailed information about getting tiny multiples started at the breast.

However the breastfeeding works out, be sure that both babies get plenty of Mom or plenty of Dad with their meals. Infant feeding is about both physical and emotional nourishment.

Bringing Multiples Home One at a Time

One baby may be ready for discharge days before the other. It will seem strange to have one baby at home and one still in the hospital. On the one hand, you get a more gradual introduction to caring for your babies at home. But on the other hand, you may find yourself stretched thin while you try to care for one baby at home and stay involved with the other one in the hospital. For a while, you may feel closer to the baby you are caring for at home. Eventually, after both have been discharged from the hospital, you will have time to reconnect with the one who was hospitalized longer, and you will be able to nurture your attachment to both babies.

There are lots of things you "should do" that you simply can't do. Do whatever you can and eliminate the "should do's" that don't apply to multiples. Get rid of the guilt that comes from feeling "I can't." You can, but differently. — Maureen Doolan Boyle, Executive Director, MOST (Mothers of Supertwins)

12

Medical Challenges for the Premature Baby

MEDICAL COMPLICATIONS CAN affect your preemie's health and create long-term challenges. Younger preemies are more likely to run into medical problems than are babies who are born closer to their due date. This chapter provides information about the most common medical challenges associated with premature birth.

The good news is that your preemie will probably never encounter most of these problems, and there is no need for you to know everything included in this chapter. In fact, reading through this chapter from start to finish may cause information overload, along with a great deal of unnecessary worry. We suggest that you read only those sections in this chapter that you need to read — the ones that describe a medical challenge your baby is already facing or complications that your doctor says are likely to occur in your preemie. You have enough to worry about right now. Don't add a bunch of what-if's to the worries that are keeping you awake at night.

RESPIRATORY DISTRESS SYNDROME (RDS)

When an infant is born prematurely, most of his organs are developed enough to handle life outside the womb, though with some difficulties. However, the lungs mature very late in gestation, and a preemie is likely to have a difficult time breathing. The most common breathing problem a preemie may encounter is respiratory distress syndrome (RDS). This was once a much more serious problem than it is today. Thankfully, medical advances have given preemies with breathing problems a much better chance at survival.

Why preemies get RDS. Inside the womb, the baby does not breathe with his lungs since he is floating in amniotic fluid. At birth, the lungs are expected to do something they have never done before: empty themselves of fluid, take a big gulp of air, absorb the oxygen from the air, and pass it into the bloodstream.

To do this job well, lungs need a substance called surfactant. Surfactant is a miraculous foamy fluid produced in the lungs. It forms a very thin coating inside the tiny air sacs (called alveoli) in the lungs. Lungs are spongy and wet, and the surfactant keeps the surfaces of the air sacs from getting too wet. Without surfactant, the air sacs are too wet to inflate well when baby inhales, and they collapse when baby exhales. When the insides of the air sacs are stuck together like a deflated wet balloon, it takes a lot of work to re-inflate them. Baby must work extra hard to inhale air into the alveoli, only to have them collapse again when he exhales. Soon his breathing becomes very labored, and most preemies don't have enough energy to keep this struggle up for very long. Soon baby is in respiratory distress.

The course of RDS varies depending on how early a baby is born. Mild RDS might cause only minimal labored breathing for a few days and then start to improve as the lungs begin producing surfactant. More severe RDS requires aggressive life-saving treatment.

How RDS is treated. A baby who is only a few weeks premature, with mild respiratory distress, may just need supplemental oxygen for a few days. Babies with moderate RDS might need continuous positive airway pressure (CPAP), puffs of air given through a mask to assist with each breath, for a while. An infant who is born very prematurely with severe RDS will probably need to be placed on a ventilator for several days or even for several weeks. He might also be given several doses of artificial surfactant. Surfactant therapy is the main reason why preemies are now able to survive when born at a very early age.

The stress of labor and postpartum life actually stimulates baby's lungs to start producing surfactant within 3 to 4 days after birth, at which point baby's breathing slowly starts to improve. Babies who have been under stress in the womb before delivery are actually born with more mature lungs and are less likely to get RDS. These stresses may include early rupture of membranes and intrauterine growth retardation. Tocolytics (medications used to delay premature labor) and steroids given to a mother in premature labor also speed up baby's lung development. If premature delivery can be held off for just a few days with tocolytics while Mom is given steroids, the baby is much less likely to develop RDS.

BRONCHOPULMONARY DYSPLASIA (BPD) AND CHRONIC LUNG DISEASE (CLD)

Infants who are treated for RDS sometimes develop a lung problem called bronchopulmonary dysplasia. Being on a ventilator, while it can be life-saving, is hard on preemie's sensitive lung tissue. Tiny scars inside the lungs (dysplasia) may form, and these may lead to a long-term decrease in lung function. Doctors refer to long-term BPD as chronic lung disease (CLD).

BPD doesn't develop in all preemies. It's more likely to occur in babies who are born very early and those who have severe RDS. It does not cause dramatic changes in baby's condition, leading to an immediate diagnosis. Instead, what usually occurs is that the respiratory distress symptoms linger longer than expected. Baby may be on the ventilator for a long time and then need to be on oxygen therapy for even longer. In older infants, the symptoms are similar to those of asthma: frequent wheezing and difficulty breathing, and breathing made even worse by a cold. Most children outgrow BPD by the time they are 2 to 3 years old, as the lungs continue to grow and the damage eventually repairs itself.

BPD-related problems are decreasing as medical advances, such as artificial surfactant and more sophisticated ventilators, are treating RDS more effectively. Here are the latest statistics on BPD:

- Infants with birth weights of 1 to 1¾ pounds (501 to 750 grams): most develop BPD and have a 75 percent chance of survival.
- Infants with birth weights of 1¾ to 2¼ pounds (751 to 1000 grams): 50 percent develop BPD and have an 85 percent chance of survival.
- Infants with birth weights of 2¼ to 3¼ pounds (1001 to 1500 grams): only about 7 percent will develop BPD and have a 96 percent chance of survival.

The best treatment for BPD is prevention. Delaying premature delivery as long as possible and treating moms in preterm labor with steroids go a long way toward reducing the incidence and severity of respiratory distress syndrome, and thus BPD. If your infant has RDS, the doctors and nurses will be constantly monitoring his progress, checking his oxygen and carbon dioxide levels, and making frequent adjustments to the ventilator settings. Their goal is to maintain baby's ventilator settings at just the right level: high enough that baby's blood carries plenty of oxygen, low enough to avoid injuring delicate lung tissue.

Most children eventually outgrow the effects of BPD, as their lungs get bigger and repair the damaged tissue. But until

baby gets bigger, you and your pediatrician will be working together to manage baby's breathing problems. Here is information about the problems associated with CLD and how to treat them.

Fatigue. Your baby may become easily fatigued and short of breath during any strenuous activity. Feeding is your baby's main form of exercise in the first few months, and he may be able to feed for just a few minutes before he needs to take a break. Signs that indicate your baby needs to rest include rapid labored breathing, flaring of the nostrils with each breath, pale or blue color around the mouth, and chest retractions (the ribs and abdomen cave in with each breath). If baby gets too fatigued too quickly with feeding, he may need to be given a little oxygen during feedings. Bouts of crying are also very tiring for babies. Do whatever you can to minimize crying. Babies with CLD should not "cry it out."

As baby starts rolling around, crawling, and eventually walking, she may experience some shortness of breath. This may slow her down a bit, but you don't need to restrict her activities. Let her do whatever she can tolerate. Through the years, her exercise tolerance may improve as her lungs grow stronger. However, some children will continue to require ongoing respiratory treatment and show lower tolerance for exercise.

Oxygen therapy. A baby or child with chronic lung disease may need to be given supplemental oxygen through nasal canula (which you are probably very familiar with by now). Babies with severe CLD may need oxygen all the time; babies with milder CLD may need oxygen only intermittently, during feedings or while sleeping. When baby was in the hospital, the oxygen monitor (pulse ox) sounded an alarm if baby's oxygen level dropped too low. Your baby's doctor may or may not recommend that you use an oxygen monitor at home. You will learn to watch baby's face as a way of monitoring her need for oxygen. If her skin is very pale or bluish in color, she probably needs oxygen.

Inhaler medications. Babies with moderate to severe CLD may need daily medications to help keep their breathing comfortable. Such medications include bronchodilators (such as albuterol) and steroids. Generally, they are delivered directly to the respiratory system using an inhaler or a nebulizer machine. (The nurses will show you how to use these before discharge.)

Diuretic medications. Some babies with severe CLD need to take daily medication that increases urine production to prevent fluid build-up in the lungs.

Fortunately, most children eventually outgrow BPD. The lungs continue to develop until about age seven, and breathing function improves as new healthy lung tissue grows around the damaged parts. Often by age 2 or 3, the lungs are fully recovered and your child may not have any lingering problems with his breathing. (See Protecting Baby's Precious Lungs, page 144, to learn how to minimize problems with CLD.)

RESPIRATORY SYNCYTIAL VIRUS (RSV)

Respiratory syncytial virus (RSV) is the most common cause of lower respiratory infection and the leading cause of hospi-

---

"IRREPARABLE DAMAGE" — NOT NECESSARILY SO!

You may at some time hear someone in the NICU use the term "irreparable damage" to describe something that has happened to your baby's lungs, intestines, or brain. We wish that caregivers would stop using this phrase. All the organs of the body have remarkable ways of repairing themselves. After all, many adults who suffer massive heart attacks go back to leading normal lives, though they may have to make significant changes in their diet and lifestyle. The younger the child, the better the chance the body has of repairing itself, since young tissue grows and regenerates at a faster pace. As you will learn throughout this book, there are many parenting and dietary "therapies," as well as medical treatments, that can help your preemie at least partially repair even the most damaged tissue.

---

talization of babies under the age of one. Around 125,000 infants in the United States are hospitalized each year with complications of RSV infection. Besides being traumatic for baby, going back into the hospital is hard on parents who have already endured weeks of NICU care. RSV is a highly contagious and potentially serious virus. Virtually all children are exposed to the RSV virus during the first two years of life and re-infection throughout life is very common. RSV is transmitted like the common cold, through close contact. Initially, the symptoms of RSV

RSV PROTECTION

The medication that is used to protect premature babies and those with heart and lung disease from RSV is the only medication that is specifically formulated for this purpose. This medicine differs from vaccines in how it builds up a baby's immunity. Most vaccines stimulate the body to produce its own antibodies against a specific disease. The RSV medication called Synagis (palivizumab) contains the actual antibodies themselves. While they do a good job of protecting high-risk children from RSV, the antibodies last only a few weeks in a baby's bloodstream. So, the shot must be given once a month for five months during the RSV season (fall through spring in most parts of the country). Synagis is a synthetically made antibody, so it is not a blood product and has few side effects.

Which preemies should get RSV shots? As of this writing, American Academy of Pediatrics guidelines state that the following infants will benefit from the RSV medication:

1. Any infant under two years of age, regardless of the degree of prematurity, with chronic lung disease.

2. Any preemie born at less than 28 weeks' gestation who is less than one year of age at the start of the RSV season.

3. Any preemie born between 28 and 32 weeks' gestation who is less than six months of age at the start of the RSV season.

4. Any preemie born between 32 and 35 weeks' gestation who has two or more risk factors, such as school-age siblings, day care exposure, or exposure to environmental air pollutants.

5. Infants with severe chronic lung disease may benefit from another round of this medication during the second RSV season.

6. Additionally, children less than two years old who have significant heart disease should also be considered.

The first RSV dose is given to high-risk children prior to their discharge from the hospital or shortly after discharge if that is during RSV season. Your baby should continue to receive a dose monthly thereafter for a total of five doses or more if the season lasts longer in your community. For updates on RSV, visit www.rsvprotection.com.

may be similar to a cold and can include fever, runny nose, coughing with difficulty breathing, difficulty eating, wheezing (a whistling sound), rapid breathing, and a blue color around the lips. An infected baby can get very sick quickly. But RSV differs from the common cold in that it moves down into the lungs and can cause wheezing and other respiratory distress. This is a concern even for full-term infants with healthy lungs, but a preemie's lungs are not as well developed and therefore much more likely to become inflamed in reaction to RSV.

Of all the infections your premature baby may catch once he or she goes home from the hospital, RSV is by far the most common and one of the most serious. The risk of serious RSV infection and hospitalization increases with risk factors such as premature birth, chronic lung disease (CLD), congenital heart disease (CHD), passive smoke exposure, day care attendance, multiple birth, family history of asthma, and birth within six months of the onset of RSV season. Since RSV complications can strike rapidly, parents of at-risk children should call their pediatrician or health care provider immediately if signs of RSV infection appear.

Babies can be protected against RSV, and all preemies with CLD or CHD should be considered for protective medication, as discussed above. (Also see Protecting Baby's Precious Lungs, page 144, to learn how to protect your baby from RSV.)

REACTIVE AIRWAY DISEASE (RAD)

Irritated airways are more likely to go into spasm. The result is wheezing. Preemies with reactive airway disease may experience wheezing for several days in response to a regular cold virus. As with RSV, inhaler medications and steroids may help reduce lung inflammation until the body fights off the virus.

RAD is a variation of asthma. Classic asthma, however, is a continuous threat; its wheezing is triggered by allergies, and it requires ongoing inhaler medication. An infant with RAD is healthy most of the time and has difficulties with wheezing only once or twice a year, when he catches a cold. The best way to minimize problems

with this condition is to prevent exposure to colds. Most infants outgrow their tendency for RAD by five years of age. (See Protecting Baby's Precious Lungs, page 144, to learn how to prevent RAD.)

AIR LEAKS

An air leak is a complication often associated with respiratory distress syndrome. When a baby is on a ventilator, air is being pushed into his lungs. A preemie's lungs are very fragile, and this air pressure can cause some of the tiny air sacs (alveoli) to burst. If enough of the alveoli burst, then air can leak out of the lungs and become trapped in other tissues in the chest cavity. This trapped air can interfere with the ability of the heart and lungs to do their job. Air leaks can also happen when an infant's own efforts to breathe are not synchronized with the ventilator. (This is why infants on ventilators are often sedated.) There are different names for this problem, depending on where the air is trapped:

- *Pneumomediastinum.* Air is trapped within the chest, but lung and heart function are not affected. This is usually mild, and it resolves without treatment.
- *Pulmonary interstitial emphysema.* Air is trapped in the supporting tissues of the lungs. This could compromise breathing by compressing the lungs.
- *Pneumopericardium.* Air is trapped in the membranes surrounding the heart. If enough air gets trapped, it can affect the pumping action of the heart.
- *Pneumothorax.* Air is trapped between the lungs and the chest wall. If baby develops a very small pneumothorax she will have only minimal difficulty breathing. A large pneumothorax causes

significant respiratory difficulty and can compress the lung on the affected side. This requires immediate, aggressive treatment.

Why air leaks happen. Air leaks can develop spontaneously in term or preterm babies when they take their first few breaths of air. These first breaths put extra pressure on the sensitive lungs. Meconium aspiration during delivery can also put extra pressure on the lungs and can lead to an air leak. (Meconium is the stool baby's body stores while in the womb. In a stressful delivery, baby's body may release this stool into the amniotic fluid, and from there it can be aspirated into the lungs.)

The term "air leak" is also used when the tube connecting baby to a ventilator does not fit snugly in his trachea and air escapes around it. This kind of air leak is simple to fix. The doctor simply substitutes a larger tube.

How air leaks are treated. Depending on its location, a small air leak may not need any treatment other than decreasing the pressure setting on the ventilator or giving baby extra oxygen.

A more significant air leak, like a large pneumothorax, needs immediate life-saving intervention. If the air collecting in baby's chest begins to interfere with heart or lung function, there may be a sudden and rapid deterioration in baby's respiratory and cardiovascular status. The lung on the affected side may collapse. The doctors can quickly diagnose the pneumothorax by listening with a stethoscope, or with a quick chest X-ray. They can insert a needle or a chest tube between baby's ribs to suction the air from the air pocket. Once the air pocket is drained, the compressed

lung expands and baby breathes more easily. The tube is left in place with suction continuing for a few days until the leaking air sacs heal. Once the alveoli heal, an air leak should not cause any long-term problems.

ANEMIA

Anemia occurs when the number of red blood cells in the blood falls below normal. Red blood cells carry oxygen to all the parts of the body. If a baby can't carry enough oxygen in his blood, he will get tired easily, won't gain weight very well, and may have difficulty breathing or coping with other medical problems.

Most premature babies become anemic at some point during their stay in the NICU. This is usually not a big problem for babies born at more than 30 weeks' gestation, and the anemia often disappears on its own. Most preemies wind up receiving iron supplements to help their body create red blood cells faster. Most babies born at 28 weeks' gestation or less need a blood transfusion to replenish their blood volume at some point during the early weeks.

Why preemies become anemic. Most babies are born with more red blood cells than they need. When they are in the womb, babies need these red blood cells to make up for the lower levels of oxygen available through the umbilical cord. Once baby is born and is breathing air, there is more oxygen available to him. He doesn't need as many red blood cells, and his body stops producing them for a while. With time, the red blood cells baby was born with naturally wear out. When the level falls below normal, baby's bone marrow begins to produce new red blood cells.

All babies go through the transition where the number of red blood cells dips and their bodies must begin to produce more. In full-term infants this happens at about 2 to 3 months of age, but in preterm infants it can be sooner, usually 4 to 8 weeks after birth. Most term babies don't have any problem producing new red blood cells, but the little body of a preterm infant, already stressed by other medical problems, can have a hard time making fresh cells. Iron is needed to make new blood, and the preemie's iron stores are much lower than a term baby's. Rapid growth and frequent blood draws increase the demand for new blood cells. Problems with bleeding in parts of the body also mean that baby must manufacture more blood.

How anemia is managed. Iron levels in the blood are measured with two tests, the hemoglobin and the hematocrit, often called an H&H. The hematocrit is the percentage of the liquid blood that is made up of red blood cells. Normal values range between 35 and 65 percent. Hemoglobin is the part of the red blood cell that carries oxygen. It usually ranges between 10 and 17 milligrams per deciliter (mg/dl). H&H numbers vary greatly depending on the age and health of the baby. They are usually higher at birth and slowly diminish over the next few months.

The neonatologist will monitor the H&H frequently, depending on how severe baby's anemia is. Some preemies can tolerate very low levels of hemoglobin without any problems and need just a small amount of iron given orally. Preemies who are fighting infection or who are on a ven-

tilator may not tolerate anemia and are more likely to need a blood transfusion. When the neonatologist is deciding if the baby needs a transfusion, he considers both the H&H numbers and baby's other symptoms. The neonatologist may also order a reticulocyte count, which indicates how quickly the baby is making new red blood cells on his own. This is another factor that influences the decision about a blood transfusion. An anemic baby's breathing, feeding, and weight gain will usually improve dramatically after a transfusion.

Give baby your blood. Many preemies need a blood transfusion at some point during their stay in the NICU. Parents may prefer to have this blood come from a family member with the same blood type as baby instead of from a blood bank. Family-member donors are called directed donors. After blood is collected from a donor, it takes approximately seventy-two hours to prepare it for transfusing. If it seems likely that your baby will need a transfusion and you prefer to use a directed donor, it is a good idea to find one early. The NICU staff will help you coordinate this. If your baby ends up not needing it, someone else will certainly benefit from the blood donation.

It is important to remember that anemia is the result of a normal process for infants; it doesn't necessarily indicate that your baby's overall condition is deteriorating. It is merely one of many roadblocks that baby must get past on his way to graduating from the NICU.

One of the latest strategies for treating anemia is a medication called erythropoietin, a hormone that occurs naturally in the body and will stimulate new blood production. Although not yet widely used, erythropoietin may become the next big breakthrough in treating anemia. Not surprisingly, breast milk contains erythropoietin — another example of the amazing properties of breast milk.

To prevent anemia in your preemie, your baby's doctor will prescribe daily iron drops for at least the first 3 to 6 months. Breastfeeding also helps to prevent anemia, since the iron in breast milk is absorbed much better than the iron in formula. If bottlefeeding, always use an iron-fortified infant formula. During your baby's routine checkups after leaving the hospital, the doctor will monitor your baby's hemoglobin level to keep anemia in check.

APNEA OF PREMATURITY

Most babies have occasional short pauses in their breathing. These pauses are termed apnea when they last for more than 15 to 20 seconds or when any pause in breathing causes baby to turn blue or causes bradycardia — a drop in heart rate to less than 100 beats per minute. (The normal heart rate for newborns is 120 to 150 beats per minute.) Episodes of apnea are very common in preemies. This is why most babies are placed on heart and breathing monitors. In fact, apnea is so common that it has nicknames: you'll hear the nurses say that a baby is having "spells," or "As and Bs" (for apnea and bradycardia). About 25 percent of all preemies who weigh less than 5 pounds 8 ounces (2500 grams) and 80 percent of those born before 30 weeks (less than 2 pounds or 1000 grams) have episodes of apnea.

Why preemies have apnea. Most apnea is related to the preemie's immature nervous system. This is called apnea of prematurity. The centers in the brain that control breathing are not fully developed, and baby occasionally "forgets" to breathe. Most babies outgrow apnea by 37 weeks' gestation. A few babies continue to have apnea spells for some months longer.

Sometimes, apnea spells indicate that a preemie is developing new medical problems, particularly if the baby starts having spells more frequently than he did before. New apnea spells can be caused by infection, anemia, low blood sugar, temperature instability, regurgitation, or even the stress of feeding.

What to do about apnea. Virtually all babies in the NICU are on heart and breathing monitors. These sound an alarm if baby has a pause in breathing or the heart rate drops too low. As soon as the alarm goes off, the nurse immediately checks on the baby to verify that the baby really has stopped breathing (often the baby is indeed breathing but has pulled one of the wire leads off his chest). These false alarms are much more common than actual apnea episodes. If the baby truly is not breathing, then the nurse calmly stimulates him by rubbing or patting his back. This is a gentle reminder to breathe. Many times, the baby starts to breathe again on her own in a few seconds without any stimulation. Rarely is a spell more severe, with the baby requiring resuscitation and oxygen to restart the breathing. Whatever it may take to get baby to breathe again, realize that apnea spells are not dangerous, though they can be scary for parents new to the NICU. Don't be put off by the nurse's laid-back attitude when it comes to spells of apnea. Keep in mind that experienced NICU nurses probably go through this routine several times per hour with the various babies they are caring for. They get very good at recognizing when a baby just needs a gentle pat to jump-start breathing, and when a baby needs some vigorous resuscitation. That's when you'll see them snap out of "mother hen" mode and become intense medical professionals.

If a preemie suddenly starts having more frequent and longer spells of apnea, the doctors usually run some basic tests to look for the problems mentioned above. If a baby continues to have frequent As and Bs, the doctors might give her a medication to stimulate breathing, such as caffeine or theophylline. If this doesn't work, continuous positive airway pressure (CPAP) can help. This treatment keeps baby breathing with a gentle constant airflow into the nose through small nasal prongs.

Going home with an apnea monitor.

Apnea spells usually disappear by the time baby is ready to go home. If a baby is still having occasional mild spells but is otherwise ready for life outside the hospital, he will go home with a monitor. While it's easy to deal with apnea while baby is being monitored in the NICU, with nurses and doctors just seconds away, taking your apnea-prone baby home, where you are the one who has to respond to the monitor, is a different story.

Be reassured. Your baby's nervous system has matured dramatically. She is now able to regulate her breathing and avoid apnea spells much better than she was a few weeks ago. If your baby was still having significant apnea spells, you wouldn't be taking her home from the hospital.

An apnea monitor is a purse-size unit with wire leads that are taped to baby's

chest. If baby stops breathing for more than twenty seconds, or if the heart rate falls below 80 beats per minute or speeds up to more than 200 beats per minute, the alarm will go off. Keep in mind that the doctors don't expect your baby to have a serious apnea episode at home. Rather, the monitor is there because there is a slight chance that your baby will have a long period of apnea that requires your attention. In this case, the alarm will sound and the noise will startle your baby and she will begin breathing again. The alarm will also call you to come to baby's aid and stimulate her to begin breathing. Before baby leaves the hospital, you will be trained in CPR in case of an emergency, but again, it is unlikely that you will ever have to use this training.

Serious apnea episodes are rare. Most episodes of apnea are short and unnoticed. In the first days of living with a monitor at home, you will probably experience many false alarms. The most common cause of false alarms is the loosening and detaching of monitor leads taped to your baby's chest. Get used to these "loose lead" alarms. They will keep you running. Every few weeks, a representative from the monitor company will come to your house and download your baby's information from the computer in the monitor. The technician will print out a record of all alarms and send this to your doctor. If any real apnea episodes occurred (longer than 20 seconds), the printout will show this.

Monitors are a mixed blessing. On the one hand, parents can rest assured that should anything happen to their baby while they are sleeping, the alarm will go off and they can come to baby's aid. On the other hand, parents can become preoccupied with the monitor. At first, your baby may be connected to the monitor twenty-four hours a day, even when awake. You will fuss all day long with the monitor leads and do your best to keep them securely attached. As the days pass, you will realize that this task is very time-consuming, and it may be interfering with your enjoyment of baby. As you become more comfortable and your doctor gives permission, you may begin to use the monitor only while baby sleeps, or when baby is left alone in another room. When baby is awake and you are attentive, you will learn to be baby's monitor. You may also find you get tired of lugging around this second "diaper bag" everywhere you go, and start leaving the monitor at home.

If a couple months go by without any real apnea episodes and you feel comfortable, your doctor may agree that you can stop using the monitor.

JAUNDICE, OR HYPERBILIRUBINEMIA

Jaundice, or hyperbilirubinemia, is the cause of the yellowish tinge that develops in a newborn's skin and eyes during the first week after birth. Jaundice is one of the more common problems in the NICU, and it is very likely that your preemie will develop jaundice to some degree. The good news is that jaundice is a simple problem, is easily treated, and seldom results in long-term complications.

Why babies get jaundice. Babies are born with excess red blood cells in their circulation. After birth, the extra red blood cells start to break down, releasing into the circulation a yellow pigment called bilirubin. The skin and the whites of the eyes develop a temporary yellow color.

The bilirubin slowly gets filtered out of the circulation by the liver and is then flushed out of the body with baby's stools. This is all a normal part of being a newborn and usually does not indicate a medical problem. Jaundice in healthy term infants usually resolves by 2 weeks of age.

Bilirubin concentrations may reach higher levels in premature infants because preemies break down their red blood cells faster and their immature livers cannot excrete the bilirubin as quickly as a full-term infant's can. Moderate increases in the bilirubin level are very common and not harmful to your baby. However, if the level of circulating bilirubin gets too high, there is a possibility that bilirubin may enter the brain, which can lead to brain damage, a condition called kernicterus. Because of careful monitoring and effective treatment of the bilirubin level, this condition is rare. Blood tests for baby's bilirubin level are part of every preemie's routine lab work during the first week or two.

Occasionally, normal newborn jaundice is exacerbated by other problems, such as mother-baby blood type incompatibility or very rare liver problems. Screening for these problems is also part of routine lab work in the NICU.

How jaundice is treated. Years ago, a nursery nurse made the observation that the newborns whose bassinets were near the windows got less jaundice. We now know that certain wavelengths of light help break down the bilirubin in the body into a form that is easier to eliminate. The modern NICU is equipped with special phototherapy lights called bililights. These look like small tanning beds, but they deliver only those wavelengths needed for bilirubin breakdown (i.e., no harmful tanning rays). During the time baby is under the lights, his eyes are covered to protect them from damage. You can ask to have the lights turned off and the eye patches removed for brief periods of time so that you and baby can enjoy some eye contact. Be sure to touch your baby and give her gentle stimulation during the time she is under the lights. There are also special biliblankets that deliver phototherapy when wrapped around baby's naked body. Eye patches are not required when using a biliblanket.

The level of bilirubin that warrants phototherapy varies according to the size and age of the baby. Younger and smaller infants usually need phototherapy sooner, at lower bilirubin concentrations. Once a baby is placed "under the lights," the bilirubin level is checked once or twice a day. The level promptly plateaus, and then starts to fall after a few days. When there is an appropriate drop in the bilirubin level, phototherapy can be stopped.

Rarely, the bilirubin level continues to increase despite phototherapy. If the level is high enough that there is a risk of brain damage, an exchange transfusion is done to get the level down quickly. In an exchange transfusion, a certain amount of blood is withdrawn from baby and replaced with an equal amount of blood from a carefully matched donor.

How high is too high? The answer depends on the baby's gestational age. Healthy full-term babies can tolerate a bilirubin level as high as 20 to 25 mg/dl, and bilirubin may not be harmful to the baby until the level reaches 25 to 30 mg/dl. Very young preemies, on the other hand, can become sick when the level reaches 20 mg/dl. Preemies are treated for jaundice long before the level gets this high.

If your infant develops jaundice and needs phototherapy, remember that this is one of the more routine problems encountered in the NICU and it need not worry you. In the case of most preemies, bililights are started early in the course of jaundice, and it is rare for a baby to need an exchange transfusion. It is also very rare for jaundice to do any permanent damage.

HEARING LOSS

Between 1 and 15 percent of babies in the NICU are affected by hearing loss (thankfully, most of these cases are mild), compared with only 0.1 percent of term babies. The delicate sound receptors in the middle ear of preemies and the nerves that carry the sound impulses from the ear to the brain are more susceptible to damage in preemies. Extremely premature infants are at greatest risk of hearing loss. Also at risk are infants who have extremely high bilirubin levels, high enough to require an exchange transfusion. (See Jaundice, or Hyperbilirubinemia, above.) Infections or bleeding in the brain can also lead to hearing loss.

How hearing loss is diagnosed. It is important to recognize hearing problems early so that appropriate treatment can be started before the hearing problems affect the child's language development. In the past, only infants with certain risk factors (very low birth weight, specific medical problems and treatments) were tested for hearing problems. Current recommendations are to screen all newborns, full-term and preemies, for hearing loss before they are discharged from the hospital.

There are several types of hearing tests for infants, but the most reliable is the Auditory Brainstem Response (ABR) test. Sensors are placed on the baby's head to measure the brain wave activity in response to noises played through earphones. This test takes about ten minutes, is painless, and is usually done while the infant is quiet or sleeping. If your baby does not pass the initial hearing screening, don't panic. The test is designed to do a good job of identifying babies who have some degree of hearing loss, and some babies with normal hearing do not pass the test. It is better to have to retest some normal babies than to miss hearing loss in others. Babies who do not pass the initial screening are referred to an audiologist for a repeat test about 1 to 3 months after the baby's original due date. Most babies pass this second test since their nervous system is more mature by this age. Babies who still do not pass need more testing to evaluate which part of the hearing system is not working.

How hearing loss is treated. If the testing confirms that your infant does not hear as well as she should, it is important . to start treatment as early as 6 months of age to minimize the effects on baby's language development. You and your baby will work with a number of specialists: an audiologist, an ear-nose-throat surgeon (ENT), and speech therapists. Potential treatments include hearing aids, cochlear implants, and possible ear tubes to prevent ear infections. You may be taught to use sign language with your baby, even if

he won't need this to communicate when he is older. Signing enhances language development even in babies who can hear normally. Technology is advancing quickly in the area of hearing loss, and new treatments should be available in the near future.

GASTROESOPHAGEAL REFLUX DISEASE (GERD)

Most preemies have some degree of gastroesophageal reflux (also known as acid reflux), which is caused by the stomach contents being regurgitated back up into the esophagus, where they may irritate its sensitive lining. Normally when we eat, the muscular band that joins the esophagus to the stomach (called the lower esophageal sphincter, or LES) contracts and closes, keeping the stomach contents in the stomach. In many infants, especially preemies, this muscular valve is immature and does not close properly. Baby's food and stomach acids leak back into the esophagus, causing something like heartburn in adults. Because of their immaturity, preemies are even more susceptible to reflux. Most infants eventually outgrow GERD between 6 and 12 months of age, but until then, reflux presents challenges to babies and their caregivers.

How Can You Tell if Your Baby Has GERD?

The severity of reflux varies greatly from baby to baby. Some preemies are "happy spitters," and the reflux doesn't seem to bother them. For these babies, reflux is more a laundry problem than a medical one. In others, reflux is so painful that it interferes with their health and growth.

Here are clues that your preemie may be suffering from reflux:

Frequent spitting up. While all babies spit up at times, babies with reflux may spit up more often, more forcefully, and more than just 1 or 2 teaspoons. (However, some preemies with GERD do not spit up at all. Their regurgitated stomach acids get only as far as the esophagus.)

Hurting while eating. One of the most common clues that a baby has reflux is the parent's observation "He acts like it hurts when he eats."

Colicky bouts of abdominal pain. Babies with GERD often arch their back, squirm, draw their legs up to their abdomen, and howl. There is no doubt that they really hurt!

Restless sleep. Regurgitation is more likely to occur when baby is in a horizontal position. Therefore, frequent night waking may be a clue that baby has reflux.

Throaty noises. Babies with GERD make unusual gagging noises during or after eating. These sounds are the result of trying to cope with spit-up in the back of the throat.

Breathing problems after eating. Preemies with severe reflux may have apnea or wheezing spells during or after a feeding.

Less reflux when upright. Babies with GERD often feed more comfortably and have less painful discomfort after feedings when they are held upright rather than laid flat.

Most reflux is diagnosed from the symptoms listed above. Sometimes a doctor may use a pH probe to determine if a baby has reflux. This is a flexible tube that is inserted through baby's mouth or nose into the esophagus, ending just above the stomach. This device measures the amount of stomach acid that is regurgitated into the esophagus over a twelve- to twenty-four-hour period.

Dr. Bob advises: Scratch the word "colic" from your vocabulary if you have a preemie. Saying "it's just colic" won't be much help to your baby. You and your doctor need to figure out what is causing the pain and the crying. We have found that the most likely cause of "colic," especially in preemies, is reflux.

Parenting the Preemie with Reflux

The basic strategy for dealing with reflux is to do whatever possible to keep the food from coming back up, while making it easier for baby's digestive system to move the food down out of the stomach and into the intestines. Try these suggestions:

1. Breastfeed. GERD is much less severe in breastfed infants. Breast milk is easier for babies to digest and empties from the stomach much faster than formula or any other food. The less time the food spends in the stomach, the less opportunity there is for regurgitation. Breastfed babies also have softer and easier-to-pass stools. Formula-fed babies are more likely to get constipated, which can aggravate reflux.

2. Use a more stomach-friendly formula. Predigested, hypoallergenic formulas (e.g., Nutramigen, Pregestimil, Alimentum, and Neocate) empty from the stomach faster than standard formulas do. Also, in some infants, reflux may be a symptom of allergy to cow's milk–based formulas.

3. Offer shorter, more frequent feedings. As a general guide, babies with severe reflux should be fed half as much but twice as often. Smaller amounts of food in the stomach are easier and faster to digest, so there is less to spit up.

4. Keep baby upright and quiet after a feeding. Let gravity help keep the food down. Hold baby upright for about thirty minutes after a feeding. Don't bounce or jostle baby after feedings, as this can aggravate reflux.

5. Burp baby more frequently. Take the time to burp the baby as you switch from one breast to the other during a feeding, or after each ounce or two of formula. When a big gas bubble is competing with food for space in the stomach, stomach contents are more likely to come back up.

6. Avoid irritating foods in your diet. In breastfed infants, sensitivity to a food in the mother's diet may aggravate reflux. Common culprits include dairy products, caffeine (coffee, tea, soda), soy products, peanuts, shellfish, chocolate, tomatoes, citrus fruits, wheat, egg whites, nuts, corn, and gassy vegetables (e.g., broccoli, cauliflower, cabbage, onions, and green peppers). Eliminate all of these foods, or just one or two at a time, from your diet for a week or two and see if it makes any difference to your baby. Dairy products are a good place to start, or any other food that you eat frequently.

7. Try a pacifier. Frequent sucking stimulates the release of saliva, which can lubricate the irritated lining of the esophagus and also act as an antacid, as well as have a calming effect on baby.

8. Find a reflux-friendly sleeping position. Discuss with your baby's doctor whether the reflux is severe enough to warrant putting baby on his side or tummy when he's sleeping. While putting infants under 6 months of age to sleep on their backs reduces the risk of SIDS, babies with severe reflux often sleep more comfortably on their tummy or left side (In this position, the gastric inlet is higher than the outlet and gravity helps keep the food in the stomach.) Never put baby to sleep on his tummy without first consulting your doctor. If baby sleeps in a crib, try elevating the head of baby's crib at least 30 degrees. Discuss with your doctor the use of a reflux wedge — a foam wedge that keeps baby's upper body elevated while sleeping. (See Reflux Wedges and Slings in Resources, page 235.) A helpful sleeping arrangement for babies with GERD (besides in your arms) is the Amby Baby Motion Bed (see page 161).

9. Try medicines for GERD. If feeding and positioning strategies don't relieve your baby's pain, and if GERD is interfering with your baby's growth and development, your doctor may decide to prescribe medication that will make baby's stomach secretions less acidic and thus less irritating to the esophagus.

10. Keep a diary. Your observations of your baby are particularly important in treating reflux. Keep a written record of what you do from feeding to feeding to relieve baby's discomfort. Keep track of what you are eating if you are breastfeeding. Note what works when and what doesn't work at all. Input from you, based on your reflux diary, will help your doctor make decisions about medication and other aspects of baby's care.

11. Enjoy support. You will get a lot of practical information by talking with other parents of preemies with reflux. The national support group for parents of children with reflux is called PAGER (Pediatric/Adolescent Gastroesophageal Reflux Association); visit their Web site at www.reflux.org.

NECROTIZING ENTEROCOLITIS (NEC)

Necrotizing enterocolitis is a serious problem that develops when a section of the intestines becomes weakened and damaged. This damage allows the bowel wall to become infected by the bacteria that are normally present in the intestines. Occasionally, the intestines may rupture, leading to a life-threatening infection within the abdomen. Very premature infants are at highest risk for NEC, especially if they require intensive life support, such as mechanical ventilation.

What causes NEC. We don't know exactly what causes NEC, and we don't know how to completely prevent it. When a baby is born very premature and needs vigorous life-saving measures, there may be times when the intestines do not receive enough oxygen-rich blood, leading to small areas of weakness in the bowel wall. Bacteria that normally live in the intestine can infect these weak areas. NEC

almost never appears before an infant has begun oral feeding. Thus, for reasons that are not clear, feeding seems to be a trigger for NEC. This is why feeding is begun very slowly in very young preemies. There is evidence that feeding babies fresh breast milk significantly lowers the risk of NEC. Breast milk that has been frozen contains lower levels of immunoprotective factors, and commercial formulas do not provide any immune protection.

Chances of developing NEC. Overall, only about 2 to 5 percent of babies in the NICU develop NEC, and most of these are the very young high-risk babies. Younger preemies with severe respiratory problems are more likely to develop NEC. Older preemies with fewer problems rarely develop NEC.

Symptoms of NEC. Common signs of NEC are bloated abdomen, vomiting, blood in the stool, and other general signs of infection, such as worsening apnea or temperature instability. Another sign of NEC is increasing amounts of milk left in the stomach between feedings (called residuals). When a preemie is started on oral feedings, the nurses watch very carefully for signs of NEC. They frequently measure the size of baby's belly, check for residuals between feedings, and check stools for blood. Most important, they give babies only small amounts of milk at first and increase these amounts very slowly.

Diagnosis and treatment of NEC. At the first sign of any intestinal difficulties, feedings are stopped for a few hours and baby is watched very carefully. If the vital signs are normal and baby does not appear ill, then a smaller feeding might be attempted.

If this is tolerated well, the difficulties are assumed to have been insignificant (e.g., a gas bubble), and regular feedings are resumed.

If it is obvious that baby is having gastrointestinal difficulties, blood work and X-rays are usually done to look for signs of NEC. If NEC is confirmed or strongly suspected, feedings are stopped and a nasogastric suction tube is placed to keep the stomach empty. Total parenteral nutrition (TPN) is given through an IV because it is very important to let the intestines rest. Antibiotics are usually started to fight the infection. Depending on the severity of the illness, frequent X-rays of the abdomen may be necessary to monitor the progression of the illness and check for intestinal rupture.

Usually within twenty-four to forty-eight hours, NEC will either get better or rapidly become worse (there seems to be no middle ground with this illness). If things are improving, then the treatments described above are usually continued for about two weeks. If all goes well, feedings are started again slowly.

Occasionally, NEC will worsen, despite treatment. If there is intestinal rupture or baby is showing life-threatening signs of shock, surgery will be done to remove the infected portion of intestine. Once the source of infection is removed, baby's condition will probably begin to improve. After the infected piece of intestine is removed, the healthy ends cannot be reattached right away. Instead, one end of the healthy intestine is attached to the surface of the skin to drain the stools. The drainage site on the skin is called an ostomy, and baby's stools empty into a plastic bag attached to the ostomy. Eventually, baby will undergo a second surgery to reattach the two ends of the intestine and will then begin to have normal bowel function.

Long-term effects of NEC. Most babies with mild NEC recover without any problems. You can expect growth, nutrition, and gastrointestinal function to be normal by the end of the first year. Babies with serious NEC may need to receive extra nutritional support for the first year or two and will probably remain small for their age. Over half of the babies who recover from serious NEC will have some degree of developmental delay as they grow older. Part of this is due to the stress and shock of the illness itself. NEC also contributes to developmental delay because it makes it difficult for a baby to get the nutrition he needs during a time of rapid brain development.

Some intestinal problems can develop as a consequence of having NEC. These affect how the gut functions and thus affect baby's ability to get nutrients from food:

• *Strictures and bowel obstruction.* Strictures are a very common complication, occurring in up to 35 percent of babies with NEC. A stricture is a section of bowel that becomes narrow as it heals after NEC. Strictures are more likely to happen in babies who have had surgery for NEC. This narrowing of a part of the intestine can cause bleeding or obstruction. A stricture will usually develop within the first two months after recovery from NEC, but sometimes it can appear as much as six months later. A bowel obstruction is a serious complication that needs prompt medical attention. Symptoms of obstruction are abdominal distention, crampy pain, severe constipation, and vomiting green bile. If a stricture is causing an obstruction, it will need to be surgically repaired.

- *Short bowel syndrome.* Babies who had a large section of bowel removed may develop a problem called short bowel syndrome (also called short gut). With part of the intestine missing, baby has difficulty digesting food and absorbing all the nutrients he needs. As he grows, the intestine will eventually learn to function normally, usually by age two. But until then, he needs extra nutritional support in the form of TPN or an elemental (predigested) formula. Babies also usually need additional calories from medium-chain triglyceride (MCT) oil (an oil that is easily absorbed from the intestines and offers a rich source of fat, calories, and extra vitamins). Baby will receive care from a pediatric gastroenterologist and a nutritionist, who understand how to maximize your baby's absorption of nutrients.

INFECTIONS

Preemies are prone to infections for a variety of reasons. A premature infant's immune system is immature and unable to fight germs effectively on its own. Because most of the protective antibodies that the baby receives from the mother are passed late in the pregnancy, a baby who is born too early misses out on this boost to the immune system. Also, many necessary life-saving medical interventions (IV lines, tubes, and catheters) can introduce germs into baby's body.

It is likely that your preemie will experience some type of infection during her stay in the NICU. Infection may be the reason she is in the NICU in the first place, since infection is a common cause of premature birth. Infections are caused by germs (viruses, bacteria, or fungi) that invade part of the body. Pneumonia is an infection in the lungs. Sepsis is an infection in the bloodstream. A urinary tract infection, or UTI, affects the bladder or kidneys. Cellulitis is an infection of the skin. Meningitis is an infection of the lining surrounding the brain or spinal cord. Infections can also occur in the bones, eyes, and most other organs.

Symptoms of an infection are usually related to the part of the body that is infected, and thus is not functioning well. Symptoms include fever, difficulty breathing, poor feeding, lethargy, or seizures. Of course, these symptoms may have causes other than infection.

Diagnosing and treating infections. If your doctor suspects that your baby has an infection, some tests will be done to pinpoint the problem. Samples of blood, urine, and spinal fluid may be sent to the laboratory for testing, and an X-ray of the chest and abdomen may be done. While waiting for the results, your infant will be started on antibiotics that are effective against a wide variety of germs. When the germs responsible for the infection are identified (usually twenty-four to forty-eight hours later), the doctors may switch to an antibiotic known to be the most effective against these specific germs. Most symptoms will improve quickly once treatment is started. Sometimes testing will not indicate the presence of a specific infection, but the doctors may choose to continue giving baby antibiotics as a precaution, in case there is an infection present that could not be identified by laboratory tests.

RETINOPATHY OF PREMATURITY (ROP)

The retina is the light-sensitive surface at the back of the eyeball. It is full of complex light receptors that are vital to normal vision. When an infant is born, the retina is still developing. Normally, tiny blood vessels begin to grow into the retina beginning around 16 weeks' gestation. These delicate capillaries grow slowly until the entire retina has a good blood supply — usually at around 32 to 34 weeks' gestation. After this, the retinal vessels continue to develop, but they are usually not vulnerable to problems. When a baby is born prematurely, the growth of the retinal capillaries is briefly interrupted.

When they start to grow again, they may grow too fast, which can lead to scarring and damage to the retina, termed retinopathy. Most of the time, the capillaries eventually slow down and grow at a normal rate, the damage heals, and vision develops normally. In more severe retinopathy of prematurity (ROP), the rapid growth continues, leading to more scarring and vision problems.

How often ROP occurs. Younger preemies are at greater risk for ROP. In babies with birth weights less than 2 pounds 3 ounces (1000 grams), or less than 28 weeks' gestation, about 90 percent will develop ROP to some degree. Many will have only a mild form and go on to develop normal vision, but some will have more serious ROP, requiring treatment. Only about 30 percent of preemies over 31 weeks develop ROP, and usually it is mild, with no long-term vision problems.

Why ROP occurs. It is still unclear why ROP develops in some preemies and not in others. Neonatologists used to think it was caused by the shock of changing from the lower oxygen concentrations of the womb to an oxygen-rich environment outside, but research has shown that ROP is more complex than that. Careful monitoring of oxygen levels in neonates has helped decrease the incidence of ROP, but it continues to be a serious problem for unknown reasons.

How ROP is treated. Infants at risk for ROP include those born at less than 31 weeks' gestation, those with birth weights less than 3 pounds 5 ounces (1500 grams), and those who have needed intensive medical interventions such as a ventilator. These infants should have their eyes examined by a pediatric ophthalmologist at about 4 to 6 weeks of age. This doctor will dilate the baby's eyes with some medicated drops and look directly at the retina for signs of ROP. If ROP is present, but only mild, then watchful waiting is the treatment, with repeat exams every 2 weeks. Most babies will get better without treatment.

If retinopathy continues to progress, treatment may be necessary at some point between 34 and 42 weeks of gestation. A small probe or laser is used to cauterize the overgrowth of blood vessels in parts of the retina in an effort to stop progression of the disease.

Vision checks throughout baby's early years. If your baby was found to have ROP, she will need one or more follow-up visits with a pediatric ophthalmologist to make sure the condition isn't worsening and to provide further treatment if necessary. If your baby does not have ROP, your doctor may suggest your preemie see the eye doctor at least once during the first year of life to make sure baby's eyes are healthy.

STRABISMUS

Strabismus is another eye condition that is more common in preemies than in full-term babies. Commonly called lazy eye, it occurs when one or more of the muscles that control eye movement is weak, preventing the eyes from moving in tandem. In the first few months of life, mild strabismus is normal, even in term babies, until the eye muscles mature. But if it persists and is left untreated, it can lead to poor vision (termed amblyopia). Your pediatrician will check closely for strabismus at well-baby checkups. If an eye doctor sees your baby for regular vision checks, he or she will also watch for any indications that baby's eyes are not consistently working together.

INTRAVENTRICULAR HEMORRHAGE (IVH)

Just as a preemie's lungs, eyes, and other body systems are fragile, so is a preemie's brain. One common complication seen in very premature babies is minor bleeding in the brain. Fortunately, this bleeding does not occur in actual brain tissue. Rather, it occurs in the ventricles, the spaces filled with spinal fluid that are located in the middle of the brain. Thus this kind of bleeding in the brain is called an intraventricular hemorrhage, or IVH. Since the ventricles are not involved in any neurologic functions, a small amount of bleeding into this space is not a problem.

However, problems can develop if there is a large amount of bleeding that leads to increased pressure in the ventricles, or if blood leaks into the brain tissue surrounding the ventricles. Intraventricular hemorrhages are classified by their severity: grades I and II are mild, while grades III and IV are more severe.

Why IVH occurs. At the bottom of the ventricles is a delicate structure called the germinal matrix, which contains some very fragile blood vessels. The trauma of premature birth and neonatal life can cause these tiny capillaries to bleed into the germinal matrix. This is a grade I hemorrhage and does not cause any problems. Further bleeding will allow small amounts of blood to leak into a ventricle: This is called a grade II IVH. A grade I or II IVH is not a problem for infants, and it will eventually resolve without any treatment. However, if there is more bleeding, the ventricle will get bigger and put pressure on the surrounding brain. This is a grade III IVH, which can lead to other problems, such as hydrocephalus (fluid in the brain; see next page) or the kind of minor brain injury associated with learning difficulties later in childhood. A grade IV IVH is much less common. It occurs when blood leaks out of an enlarged ventricle and into the surrounding brain tissue. It is the worst type of IVH and is very likely to injure the brain.

How often IVH occurs. Over the years, improvements in neonatal care have lowered the incidence of IVH. About 20 to 30 percent of infants with birth weights less than 3 pounds 5 ounces (1500 grams) will experience some form of IVH. Around 5 percent of these infants will have a grade

III or IV IVH. In infants born at less than 25 weeks' gestation, 16 percent will have a grade III or IV IVH; the incidence of grade III or IV IVH is only 2 percent in infants born after 25 weeks' gestation. About 50 percent of brain bleeds happen within the first six to twelve hours of life, and 90 percent happen in the first three days of life.

How IVH is treated. The main treatment for IVH is prevention, and many of the medications that are used to treat preterm labor also decrease the chances of IVH in preemies. Since high blood pressure increases the risk of IVH, the NICU team works very hard to avoid large fluctuations in the baby's blood pressure or blood electrolytes in the first days after birth. Giving sedation to preemies who are agitated is another strategy for preventing IVH.

In the first week to ten days, most NICUs screen all preemies under 3 pounds 5 ounces (1500 grams) for IVH with an ultrasound of the brain. Older infants who are very sick may also be screened. The ultrasound is a gentle and noninvasive test. (You're probably familiar with ultrasound from your pregnancy.) Your baby will most likely sleep through it.

If a brain bleed is detected, there is no special treatment to make it stop. Fortunately, most bleeds stop quickly on their own and do not cause any problems. Larger bleeds can cause pressure inside the ventricles and may lead to other problems such as anemia, seizures, apnea and bradycardia, and hydrocephalus. Various treatments and medications can be used to deal with these complications.

Even a large IVH will eventually stop bleeding. As the extra fluid is reabsorbed, the swelling of the ventricles may resolve without causing any long-term damage. More extensive bleeding can compromise brain function, affecting hearing, vision, strength, and coordination, and can also lead to learning disabilities.

HYDROCEPHALUS

Hydrocephalus literally means, "water in the head." The "water" in hydrocephalus is actually spinal fluid. The brain is constantly producing spinal fluid, which then circulates through the ventricles (cavities in the middle of the brain), the spinal cord, and the surface of the brain. This fluid is eventually absorbed into the bloodstream. Any imbalance in production or reabsorption of the fluid, or an obstruction in its flow, can cause a buildup of fluid within the ventricles. This is a process that happens very slowly and causes the ventricles to enlarge. Baby's head must grow to accommodate the extra fluid, and a head that is growing too fast can be the first sign of hydrocephalus. The enlarged ventricles can put pressure on the surrounding brain, leading to a variety of symptoms, such as apnea, irritability, or lethargy.

Why hydrocephalus occurs. Approximately one-third of neonatal hydrocephalus is caused by a genetically inherited condition in which the aqueduct that connects the ventricles is too narrow, leading to a buildup of fluid and pressure within the ventricles. More commonly, hydrocephalus is a result of intraventricular hemorrhage (see page 202) or other injury to the brain during the vulnerable neonatal period.

How hydrocephalus is diagnosed. Usually the first sign of hydrocephalus is that baby's head is growing too fast. This rapid growth may not be evident until several months after baby comes home from the NICU. While baby is in the NICU, his head will be measured, and the measurements will be plotted on a growth chart (see sample chart on page 219). If baby's head is growing too quickly, the doctor may order an ultrasound to check the size of the ventricles. Just like the ultrasound done during your pregnancy, this test is quick and painless. If the ultrasound indicates that baby has hydrocephalus, the doctors will probably use an MRI to get more information about the specific area of obstruction.

How hydrocephalus is treated. If the hydrocephalus is mild and your child does not have any symptoms, the problem may resolve itself within a few months. The doctors may decide simply to keep a watchful eye on baby's head growth and repeat the ultrasound at intervals to be sure the problem is not getting worse.

If the hydrocephalus continues to worsen, then treatment may be necessary. If the cause is an overproduction of fluid, medication may be used to decrease the production of spinal fluid. If there is a blockage somewhere in the system, the excess fluid is drained into the abdomen by a ventriculoperitoneal (VP) shunt. A neurosurgeon places one end of a tiny flexible tube into the enlarged ventricle. The other end of the tube goes into baby's abdomen, where the excess fluid is reabsorbed. In between, the tube travels under baby's skin, where it is hardly noticeable. Placing a VP shunt may sound difficult, but it is actually one of the easier procedures that a highly skilled neurosurgeon performs. As your child grows, he may

occasionally need to have his shunt replaced simply because he is getting bigger. Your child may need 2 or 3 shunt revisions during his childhood.

Long-term effects of hydrocephalus and a VP shunt. Most children with hydrocephalus, with or without a shunt, grow and develop right alongside their peers and have normal brain function. In some infants, however, hydrocephalus combined with other medical problems creates developmental challenges. These infants may be a little slower to reach such developmental milestones as walking and talking. They may need some special educational services and physical therapy during early childhood to help them reach their full potential. It is important that development be monitored closely so that any problems are recognized and treated early. (For more on the first year at home and Early Intervention Programs, see page 174.)

Home care for a child with a VP shunt. If your child has a VP shunt, be sure you are familiar with how the shunt works. Ideally, the doctor can show you a sample of the shunt and demonstrate its various parts. Be sure you know if there is an on/off control valve that might accidentally get turned off. Keep the name and model of the shunt with your child's medical records. Above all, you need to be familiar with the signs of shunt malfunction. VP shunts are usually very reliable, but they can occasionally malfunction, allowing pressure to build up in the head again. A shunt malfunction is usually caused by obstruction or infection. Flow through the shunt can be totally or partially blocked by blood, tissue, bacteria, or a "kink" in the tube. Depending on the location of the blockage, part or all of the shunt may need to be replaced.

Signs of shunt infection. Shunt infections are usually caused by bacteria that are normally present in the body. A child does not "catch" a shunt infection if he is exposed to another child with an illness. Treating a shunt infection usually requires intravenous antibiotics and/or replacement of the infected shunt. Anytime your child has a fever with no obvious cause (such as cough, cold, sore throat, or ear infection), your neurosurgeon should be contacted to determine whether the shunt should be checked for infection. Whenever your child is being treated for an illness, be sure to remind your pediatrician that he or she has a VP shunt.

Signs of VP shunt obstruction. The increased pressure inside the head caused by a malfunctioning shunt can cause brain damage. It is important to recognize the signs of obstruction early:

- a bulging fontanel (the soft spot on top of the head)
- swelling or increasingly visible veins in the scalp
- redness or swelling of the skin along the shunt line
- unexplained lethargy or irritability
- seizures
- persistent vomiting
- in an older child, headaches, vision problems, or difficulty concentrating; you may notice changes in behavior, coordination, balance, sleep, or school performance

CEREBRAL PALSY (CP)

Cerebral palsy is the result of damage to the brain before or during birth. The nerves and muscles linked to the injured part of the brain do not work well. CP may be mild and barely noticeable, or there may be more severe weakness of the arms, legs, or facial muscles that interferes with walking or other normal activities. CP virtually never affects mild or moderately premature babies. Extremely premature babies, however, do have a slight chance of developing CP. Studies have shown that babies born at less than 1000 grams (about 2 pounds 3 ounces) have about a 10 percent chance of developing varying degrees of CP. Micropreemies (less than 26 weeks at birth and weighing less than 750 grams, or 1½ pounds) have only a 20 percent rate of cerebral palsy.

Mild CP is difficult to detect in the early months of life. It becomes more apparent as a baby grows and does not meet expected milestones in motor development or the muscles in the arms or legs become noticeably stiffer. Sometimes it's so mild that it may take years to be identified. The parent or pediatrician is usually the first person to suspect CP. The diagnosis will be confirmed by a neurologist, and therapy will be provided by an occupational therapist to help baby overcome any difficulties.

HERNIA

Premature baby boys are more likely to develop a hernia than their full-term buddies are. Around 32 weeks' gestation, the testicles move from inside the abdomen down into the scrotum through a small tunnel in the abdominal muscles. Pressure in baby's abdomen may also push fluid and part of the intestines down into this tunnel. This makes a bulge in the scrotum. Babies who stay in the womb long enough don't have this abdominal pressure, so hernias are very rare in full-term infants. Preemie girls may also develop hernias, though not as often as boys do. You will see a bulge to the side of the vagina in girls. The hernia may appear while baby is in the NICU, but more often it will show up after baby has gone home. If you notice a bulge, don't panic. Just show it to your doctor at the next checkup (or right away if it seems to be hurting baby). Repairing an inguinal hernia, as this is called, requires a minor surgical procedure when baby is around six months old.

Another type of hernia, an umbilical hernia, may appear on baby's tummy. You may notice that your baby's belly button bulges out like a little balloon when he cries. Baby's abdominal muscles have not yet grown together around the belly button, and the abdominal pressure that goes along with crying pushes out against baby's skin. Nearly all of these resolve on their own, but it may take a few years. If there is still a large bulge after age five, a minor surgical procedure can correct it.

PATENT DUCTUS ARTERIOSUS (PDA)

While in the womb, a baby receives oxygen from his mother through the placenta. Since there is no need for the blood to travel to the lungs to pick up oxygen, the blood bypasses the lungs, following the path of a blood vessel called the ductus arteriosus (sometimes just called the ductus). In the first day after baby's birth, the ductus closes on its own, allowing blood to flow into the lungs to pick up oxygen, then back to the heart and out to the rest of the body.

In premature infants, the ductus tends to stay open, and some of the blood continues to bypass the lungs, circulating out to the body without picking up vital oxygen. This is called a patent (open) ductus arteriosus, or PDA. This is a common problem in very young preemies, occurring in about 45 percent of infants under 1750 grams (about 3 pounds 14 ounces) and almost 80 percent of infants under 1000 grams (about 2 pounds 3 ounces). For the first few days, a preemie with a PDA will probably need a little more oxygen than usual (which he would probably need even without the PDA, because his lungs are immature), but the PDA doesn't affect the function of the heart and lungs significantly. However, over the next few days or weeks, this extra blood flow can put a strain on the heart and lungs. If it is allowed to continue, the heart can tire out, resulting in a condition called congestive heart failure (CHF). A PDA can also lead to pulmonary edema, in which fluid from the blood leaks into the tissues of the lungs, making it more difficult for baby to breathe. The severity of the problems caused by a PDA depends on how much blood is flowing through it. Small PDAs cause only minor problems and may close eventually on their own. A large PDA will probably remain open and need treatment before it causes significant problems.

How PDA is treated. If the doctors suspect your baby has a PDA, their suspicions can be confirmed with an ultrasound of the heart, called an echocardiogram (or echo for short). This test is painless, and is usually done while your infant is resting. Small PDAs are easily treated with an aspirinlike medication called indomethacin. This will help the ductus to close after one or more doses. The doctors might also reduce your baby's fluid intake and give her a diuretic to get rid of extra fluid. This will reduce the amount of work done by the heart and prevent heart failure. If the indomethacin does not work, or if the medication cannot be used because of baby's other medical problems, then the ductus may need to be closed surgically. The surgeon will tie off the ductus through a small incision in your baby's chest, a procedure that takes about an hour. Although surgery on an infant can be scary for parents to contemplate, be assured that PDA surgery is routine and very safe. Once the PDA is fixed, there are no long-term effects to worry about.

SEIZURES

Seizures (involuntary twitching or muscle spasms in the face or extremities) are not uncommon in preemies. There are several medical problems that can trigger seizures, but some preemies will experience seizures for no apparent reason except that their nervous system is immature. If your baby does have one or more seizures, the medical team will do a number of tests to look for the reason. These are the most common causes of seizures:

- *Low blood sugar.* This condition is easily evaluated with a quick blood test.
- *Mineral imbalances in the bloodstream.* A blood test for calcium, magnesium, sodium, and other mineral levels will determine if this is the cause of the seizures.
- *Infection.* An infection in the bloodstream or within the brain can trigger seizures. If the doctor suspects an infection, he or she will order blood tests and may do a spinal tap.
- *Bleeding in the brain.* This can occur in young preemies and will be evaluated with an ultrasound of the brain (see Intraventricular Hemorrhage, page 202).

Besides looking for the cause of the seizures, the doctor may also order an Electroencephalogram (EEG) in order to determine the type of seizure activity that is occurring within the brain. Monitor wires are taped to baby's scalp, and the electrical activity in the brain is measured. The EEG will show if any part of the brain is experiencing an overload of electrical activity that is triggering the seizure.

There are generally two different types of seizures: those with a medical cause (such as those listed above), and those without an identifiable medical cause. If a medical cause for the seizure is quickly found and treated, then the seizures usually resolve with little or no seizure medication. If, however, the doctors can't find a cause, and the seizures continue to occur, baby will likely be treated with a medication called phenobarbital. This drug has been used for many decades and is very safe. Your baby will most likely outgrow the seizures during the first year of life.

SUDDEN INFANT DEATH SYNDROME (SIDS)

In light of new research, SIDS should no longer be considered a mysterious cloud that hangs over cribs and causes babies to take their last breath. Because of new insights into ways to lower the risk of SIDS, in recent years the incidence of SIDS has decreased by around 50 percent. Armed with a new understanding of SIDS, parents can at least do something to reduce their worry and reduce the risk. SIDS seems to be caused by a combination of many factors: immature development of cardiorespiratory control mechanisms, defective arousability from sleep in response to breathing difficulties, medical conditions that compromise breathing, and unsafe sleeping practices. Therefore, suggestions for reducing the risk of SIDS address these factors.

1. Place babies to sleep on their backs.

The "Back to Sleep" campaigns in many countries have decreased the risk of SIDS by as much as 50 percent. The main reason why back-sleeping lowers the risk is that a baby's arousability from sleep — an infant's built-in protective mechanism — works better when she sleeps on her back. Also, a baby sleeping facedown may press her head into the mattress, forming a pocket of air around her face. When this occurs, she then rebreathes exhaled air, which has diminished oxygen.

2. Use safe sleeping environments.

Avoid putting baby to sleep on unsafe surfaces, such as beanbags or couches. If using a crib, be sure the crib meets the safety standards of the Juvenile Products Manufacturers Association (JPMA). If sleeping with your baby, be sure to follow the safe-cosleeping tips listed on page 160.

3. No smoking, please! Studies show
that exposure to cigarette smoke increases

the risk of SIDS from three to five times, depending on the amount of exposure. Even exposure to secondhand smoke can increase the risk of SIDS.

Suppose you were about to take your baby into a room, when you noticed the following sign posted on the door: WARNING! THIS ROOM CONTAINS POISONOUS GASES THAT HAVE BEEN LINKED TO CANCER, LUNG DAMAGE, AND SUDDEN INFANT DEATH SYNDROME (SIDS), AND ARE ESPECIALLY HARMFUL TO THE BREATHING PASSAGES OF YOUNG INFANTS. You certainly wouldn't take your baby in there! But that's exactly what happens when your baby spends time in a room frequented by smokers. Smoke interferes with the development of the cardiorespiratory control centers in a baby's brain. In addition, smoke paralyzes the cilia — tiny filaments that line the air passages of the lungs and clear away excess mucus, which can compromise a baby's breathing. Also, mothers who smoke have lower levels of prolactin, the hormone that regulates milk production. Prolactin deficiency may lead to diminished maternal awareness of, and responsiveness to, an infant's needs.

4. Breastfeed your baby. Breastfeeding
seems to lower the risk of SIDS because of the three M's: the milk, the method, and the mother. Breast milk is kinder to tiny airways because it doesn't contain the allergens that may be present in formula. Breastfeeding reduces gastroesophageal reflux, which may cause stop-breathing episodes. The act of breastfeeding seems to improve a baby's breathing and swallowing coordination. By increasing a mother's intuition hormones, breastfeeding also increases a mother's awareness of her baby, especially during sleep. A 2004

study reported in the *Archives of Diseases of Childhood* showed that arousability from sleep — thought to be the most important SIDS risk-reducing factor — is greater in breastfed infants than in formula-fed infants. While breastfeeding is not often included in the list of major SIDS risk-reducing practices, when you put all the benefits of breastfeeding together, you have a compelling case that breastfeeding increases an infant's chances of health and well-being.

For more detailed and updated information on SIDS risk-reducing factors, see www.AskDrSears.com/SIDS. Also see *SIDS: A Parent's Guide to Understanding and Preventing Sudden Infant Death Syndrome,* by William Sears (Little, Brown, 1995).

IF YOUR BABY DIES — GRIEVING

When a baby dies in the NICU, obviously, tremendous grief is felt by the family and the medical team. Great amounts of emotional and physical energy are invested in each preemie, and it is a terrible tragedy when the story doesn't end well. Many parents of preemies who have died shared their thoughts with us. Here are some suggestions that they found particularly helpful in their grieving process.

Be with your baby, even hold him, while he is dying. You probably feel like you can't handle watching your baby die, but parents who have been through this say that it was very important for them to do this. If fact, some parents have shared with us that they criticized themselves later for choosing not to be with their baby while he was dying. If you stay with your baby, holding and comforting him, you will know that you did everything possible to make his short life full of love. A common scenario is that after weeks of high-tech intensive care with lots of noisy machines and tubes attached to your baby, it becomes clear that the battle is lost, and the decision to withdraw life support is made. This can be a peaceful time, with no beeping monitor alarms, for saying good-bye. Some parents have felt a sense of relief to see their baby finally at peace, since baby had such a struggle during his stay in the NICU.

Collect some mementos of your baby. While you might be too grief stricken at first to think about keeping some of your baby's things, it is important to salvage what you can. Eventually, maybe weeks or months later, you will realize how meaningful these things can be. A picture, a hat, or a stuffed animal from his incubator will help keep his memory alive. If you need to, ask a friend or one of the nurses to collect some things for you. Even if your child's life was brief, the memories of his life will last forever, and having some tangible items may be very important to you in the future.

Be sure he has a name. Even if your baby doesn't survive more than a few hours after his premature birth, it is important that he have a name. This will help give your baby an identity, and it will be comforting to you when loved ones refer to him by name. "A few months ago, my wife's third pregnancy ended with a late miscarriage, and we have since found it very meaningful to use the baby's name when we talk about him," says Dr. Jim.

Invite friends and family to the funeral. Even though most of the people in your life never got a chance to meet your baby, you will find it comforting to have your loved ones with you during this time. The funeral will be a good time for public recognition of your baby's life. Sharing the memories of your child's life with some friends and family will help you acknowledge what has been lost and allow you to mourn openly and fully.

What about an autopsy? You will probably be asked if an autopsy can be performed. You can decide against this if you wish, and if you are not sure, ask for more time before making a decision. Here are a few issues to consider in your decision. An autopsy can give you some definite answers about why your child died. This can be helpful to you in the future in giving you a sense of closure. Also, the information gained from autopsies has helped doctors better understand the problems of prematurity and has led to better care for preemies. Parents often feel good about helping preemies in the future. An autopsy will not disfigure your baby, and you can still have an open-casket funeral if you wish. The autopsy can also be done very quickly and should not interfere with the planning of the funeral.

Managing Your Grief

Wounds heal. Life goes on. Scars remain. To grieve in a healthy way, maintaining a healthy connection with your infant while dealing with the loss, you need to call upon many resources, both personal and professional, for help. While there is no magic formula that fits everyone, there are time-tested ways of growing while grieving that many parents have found useful.

Get into your grief, not out of it. After losing a child, people are often urged to keep busy, to immerse themselves in their work, to have another baby quickly — to escape the grief somehow. This usually doesn't work. Your baby will always be part of your life, and you must acknowledge this fully or the hurt will continue to fester underneath a controlled facade. Healthy grieving means getting in touch with your feelings, mourning as you need to mourn, and learning to live with memories that still live in your home.

Take good physical care of yourself. Remember, grieving depresses the mind and the body. You may not want to eat, drink, or exercise, but you need to. Be sure to drink a lot of fluids to keep yourself from getting dehydrated, as dehydration aggravates depression. You may have to force yourself into an exercise routine, perhaps the ritual of a half-hour morning walk. Exercise will help your daily mood. Depression diminishes your appetite, but you owe it to yourself to nourish your body.

Express your grief. Use your talents to handle grief. If you have musical talent, compose songs. If you have a flair for writing, compose poems. Poems can be very therapeutic for the writer and the listener, especially during hard times or on special days, when grief may be more difficult to handle.

Get help. Seek the comfort of family and friends, or get professional help if you need to. Support groups are available, and the NICU staff probably have some local connections for you. A number of books are solely devoted to dealing with the loss of a baby. One such title is *Empty Cradle, Broken Heart: Surviving the Death of Your Baby* (Fulcrum Publishing, 1996), by Deborah L. Davis. Another good resource is SHARE Pregnancy and Infant Loss Support, Inc. Visit www.nationalshareoffice.com.

Appendix 1: Weight Conversion Table

this weight in grams	equals	this weight in pounds and ounces
680 g		1 lb 8 oz
737 g		1 lb 10 oz
794 g		1 lb 12 oz
851 g		1 lb 14 oz
907 g		2 lbs
964 g		2 lb 2 oz
1 kilogram 1021 g		2 lb 4 oz
1077 g		2 lb 6 oz
1134 g		2 lb 8 oz
1191 g		2 lb 10 oz
1247 g		2 lb 12 oz
1304 g		2 lb 14 oz
1361 g		3 lbs
1418 g		3 lb 2 oz
1474 g		3 lb 4 oz
1531 g		3 lb 6 oz
1588 g		3 lb 8 oz
1644 g		3 lb 10 oz
1701 g		3 lb 12 oz
1758 g		3 lb 14 oz
1814 g		4 lbs
1871 g		4 lb 2 oz
1928 g		4 lb 4 oz
1985 g		4 lb 6 oz
2 kilograms 2041 g		4 lb 8 oz
2098 g		4 lb 10 oz
2155 g		4 lb 12 oz
2211 g		4 lb 14 oz
2268 g		5 lbs
2325 g		5 lb 2 oz
2381 g		5 lb 4 oz
2438 g		5 lb 6 oz
2500 g		5 lb 8 oz

Appendix 2: Discharge Resources

WHEN YOUR BABY is discharged from the hospital, you may be given some follow-up appointments with various medical specialists. You will also be given several phone numbers for resources, such as a home health equipment company, community resources for preemies, and hospital follow-up clinics. Instead of trying to keep track of all these appointments and phone numbers separately, here is a place where you can conveniently write down everything you need for your baby's follow-up.

DISCHARGE INSTRUCTIONS AND MEDICATIONS

_____

_____

_____

_____

_____

_____

CONTACTS AND APPOINTMENTS

NICU (in case you have questions once you're home — and you will!)

Your primary nurse's name _____ Phone no. _____

Pediatrician's name _____ Phone no. _____

Follow-up appointment _____

Neonatologist's name _____ Phone no. _____

Follow-up appointment _____

Lactation consultant's name _____ Phone no. _____

Follow-up appointment _____

Apnea monitor company name _____

Phone no. _____ Follow-up appointment _____

Other home health company name _____

Phone no. _____

Other medical specialists (neurologist, neurosurgeon, cardiologist, gastroenterologist, etc.)

Name _____ Specialty _____

Phone no. _____ Appointment _____

Name _____ Specialty _____

Phone no. _____ Appointment _____

Name _____ Specialty _____

Phone no. _____ Appointment _____

Early Intervention Program _____ Name _____

Phone no. _____ Appointment _____

OTHER RESOURCES

Name _____ Phone no. _____

Name _____ Phone no. _____

Name _____ Phone no. _____

Appendix 3:
Plotting Your Preemie's Growth in the NICU

ON PAGE 219 is a standard preemie growth chart. You can track your baby's weight, length, and head circumference as he grows over the weeks and months. Start by plotting these measurements at the date of birth. For example, if your baby was born at 30 weeks' gestation, plot your baby on the 30-week line and continue week by week from there. Your nurse will also be plotting these measurements on a similar graph in baby's chart. Ask your nurse to show you where this record is kept so you can refer to it.

How does your baby's size compare to that of other babies? We use three terms to describe a preemie's size:

Appropriate for gestational age (AGA). This means that a baby's weight is similar to that of most babies born at the same gestational age. For example, according to the graph, a 32-week preemie would typically weigh between 1300 and 2100 grams. Therefore, any 32-week preemie who weighs within this range is thought to have an appropriate weight.

Small for gestational age (SGA). If your preemie's weight is below the growth curve at the time of birth, then he is considered small for his gestational age. For example, a 32-week preemie who weighs 1200 grams or less at birth would be considered SGA.

Large for gestational age (LGA). If your preemie's birth weight is above the growth curve, then he is considered large for his gestational age. For example, a 32-week preemie weighing more than 2200 grams at birth is larger than expected. This may mean that baby will experience fewer preemie complications and leave the NICU sooner than expected. But predictability is not a word used in the NICU.

Percentiles. As your baby grows, you will notice he grows along a certain percentile line. This line compares your baby's size to that of other babies at each week of gestational age. For example, a 32-week preemie who is 44 centimeters long is on the 75th percentile line. This means he is longer than 75 percent of other 32-week preemies.

The percentile at any one week is not very significant. What the medical team will be watching is baby's growth trend over several weeks and months. They want to make sure baby's weight, length, and head circumference are gaining steadily and consistently. Too much or too little growth in any of these areas can indicate a nutritional or medical problem that requires attention.

Classification of Newborns (Both Sexes) by Intrauterine Growth and Gestational Age

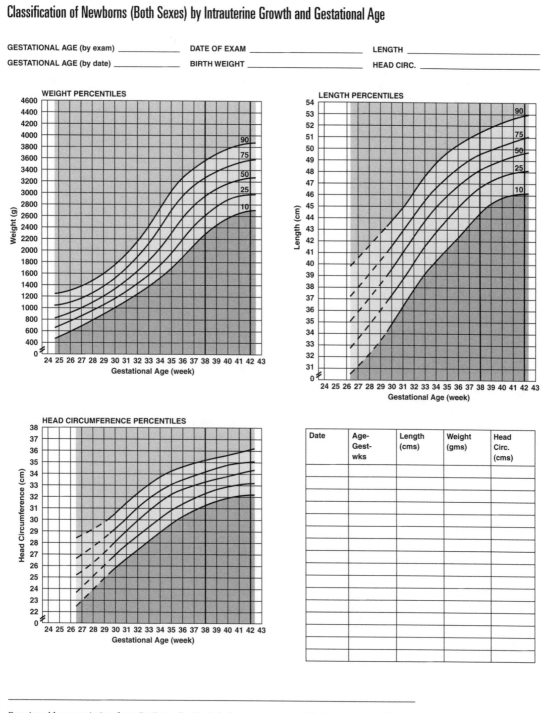

GESTATIONAL AGE (by exam) _____   DATE OF EXAM _____   LENGTH _____

GESTATIONAL AGE (by date) _____   BIRTH WEIGHT _____   HEAD CIRC. _____

Reprinted by permission from Dr. Battaglia, Dr. Lubchenco, *Journal of Pediatrics* and *Pediatrics*.

Appendix 4:
Plotting Your Baby's Growth Through the First Year

ON PAGE 223 is a growth chart for a girl from birth to 36 months. This is the same chart that your pediatrician will use to plot your baby's growth during your regular checkups. We have added dots to show how this would be done for a preemie who was born 3 months early (28 weeks):

- At 2 months of chronological age, your baby weighs 6½ pounds. Your pediatrician plots this on the 2-month line. Notice that this weight is far below the normal growth curve for a full-term baby. But if we consider that baby's corrected gestational age (CGA) is actually 36 weeks (one month before the full-term due date), then baby is actually about average weight. This adjustment is indicated by the arrow pointing back 3 months to baby's CGA.
- At 4 months, baby weighs 9¼ pounds, still below the normal growth curve. Correcting for 3 months of prematurity, baby's CGA would be 1 month. Compared with full-term 1-month-old babies,

her weight is on the 50th percentile line. This means she weighs more than 50 percent of 1-month-old babies. This is an average weight.
- At 6 months, baby weighs 11½ pounds. Correcting back 3 months, her weight is on the 25th percentile line compared with other 3-month-old babies. This means that she weighs more than 25 percent (and less than 75 percent) of babies at this age, a slightly below-average weight, but still healthy.
- At 9 months, baby weighs 15½ pounds, now just barely on the growth curve for her chronological age. Correcting back 3 months, she is approximately on the 40th percentile line. She has gained weight slightly faster than in the previous 3 months.
- At 12 months, baby weighs 18 pounds. She is now on the 10th percentile line of the growth chart if we don't correct back 3 months and compare her weight with other one-year-old babies. Correcting back 3 months, she is on the 35th percentile line.

• At some point between age one and two years, your doctor will stop correcting back for the 3 months of prematurity and simply plot your baby's weight according to her chronological age.

Your pediatrician will plot your baby's length (on the same graph) and head circumference (graph not included here) in a similar manner. You can obtain growth charts online at www.cdc.gov/growthcharts or from your pediatrician.

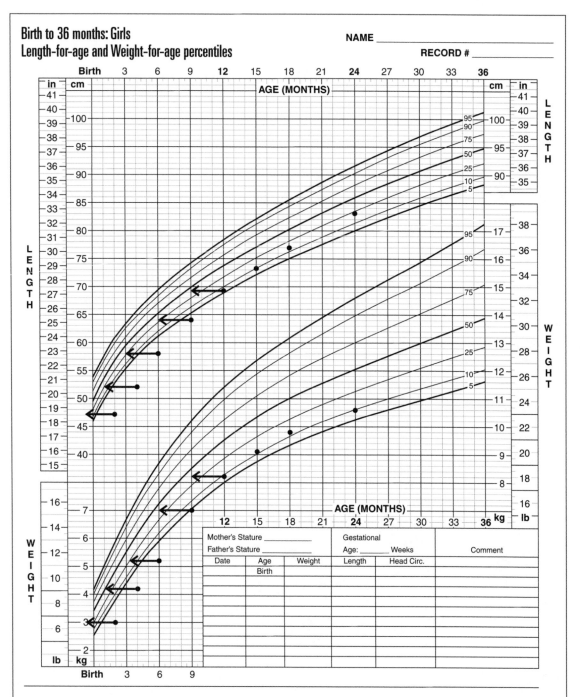

Birth to 36 months: Girls
Length-for-age and Weight-for-age percentiles

NAME _____

RECORD # _____

Published May 30, 2000 (modified 4/20/01)
SOURCE: Developed by the National Center for Health Statistics in collaboration with
the National Center for Chronic Disease Prevention and Health Promotion (2000).

Appendix 5:
Newborn and Infant CPR

BELOW ARE THE BASICS of infant CPR. All parents and caregivers should take the CPR class offered at your NICU.

Be sure to ask your neonatologist if there are any special CPR modifications you need to know for *your* baby.

Step one: Quick assessment. If baby is pale, blue, and obviously not breathing, begin CPR, as in step two, immediately. If you are uncertain, look, listen, and feel for breathing.

Step two: Clear the mouth. Look for foreign objects, food, or gum. Carefully remove anything you find with a visible, not a blind, finger sweep. If there is vomit or any other fluid in the mouth, turn your child on one side and use gravity to clear it. If you suspect choking, apply back blows.

Step three: Position baby to straighten the airway. Place baby on his back, his head level with his heart. Place one hand on his head and your fingers on his chin. Clear the tongue from the back of the throat by lifting the chin up with one hand while pressing on the forehead with the other.

An infant's head should be slightly tilted upward toward the ceiling (called the sniffing position — do a practice sniff and notice how your head moves slightly upward and forward). Do not tilt an infant's head as far back as you would an adult's, as this may obstruct the airway. A towel rolled up under the neck usually maintains the correct position.

Step four: Begin mouth-to-mouth breathing. Cover the baby's *mouth and nose* with your mouth. Blow into baby's mouth with just enough force to see baby's chest rise. (Blow with just the air in your cheeks, more a *puff* than a breath, not with the full force of a deep breath during exhaling. Forcing too much air in too fast may damage baby's lungs or distend the stomach and compromise breathing or trigger vomiting.) Begin with two short breaths. Watch for a chest rise during your blow.

If baby's chest rises, you know the airway is clear and your technique is right. Continue mouth-to-mouth blowing until your baby is breathing on his own. Give a steady breath every three seconds (twenty per minute).

Step five: Check baby's pulse. If you feel a pulse, it means baby's heart is beating and you do not have to pump on baby's chest. The easiest way to find a pulse in a baby is by pressing gently between the muscles on the inner side of the upper arm, midway between the shoulder and the elbow. An alternate site in a child is the side of the neck. Most CPR in tiny babies requires only breathing help, not chest compressions. If baby has no pulse, go on to step six.

Step six: Begin chest compressions. Place baby on a firm surface, such as the floor or a table. Open or remove baby's shirt. Place two or three fingers on the breastbone just below the nipple line (or use the two-thumb method shown in the illustration below). Depress the breastbone (the heart is right underneath) to a depth of one-half to one inch (1½ to 2½ centimeters) and at a rate of *at least one hundred per minute* — easy to time by counting "one and two and one and two and . . . ," saying "and" during the release and the number while depressing the sternum in a smooth, nonjerky rhythm.

If you are doing CPR by yourself, give baby a blow of mouth-to-mouth air after every fifth heart compression, being sure to maintain proper head position, and watch for baby's chest rising. Do not lift your fingers off the skin between strokes, except to do mouth-to-mouth breathing.

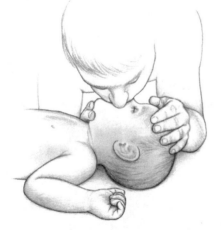

Mouth-to-mouth breathing for infants under one year.

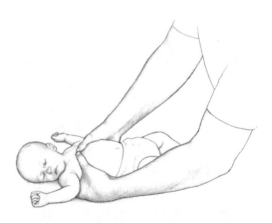

Chest compression of newborn.

In review, the ABC's* of CPR are:

- **A — airway:** Position baby's head and remove obstructions to clear the airway.
- **B — breathing:** Do mouth-to-nose-and-mouth breathing with baby's head properly positioned and at a rate of one breath every three seconds.
- **C — circulation:** If you do not feel a pulse or heartbeat, do chest compressions at one hundred strokes per minute.
- **D — dial 911:** Call for help whenever it's practical, within a minute or two of starting CPR.

---

* The procedures for treating choking and administering CPR are those currently recommended by the American Academy of Pediatrics. New research periodically alters these recommendations, so refresher courses are necessary to learn updated techniques. (For updates see www.AskDrSears.com.)

Glossary of Medical Terms

URING YOUR WEEKS in the NICU, you will hear nurses, doctors, and other medical personnel use many unfamiliar terms. When you hear something you don't understand, a staff member will be more than happy to pause and explain it to you. This glossary will provide you with another means to understand any medical jargon that flies past you. You may wish to read through these terms during the first days of baby's stay in the NICU and then refer back to them when you hear them mentioned again.

ABG. Arterial blood gas. See blood gas.

ABO incompatibility. ABO refers to blood type. In certain cases, when a baby's blood type differs from the mother's, this can lead to increased jaundice.

ABR. Auditory brain stem response. A specialized hearing test.

AGA. Appropriate for gestational age. This means baby's birth weight was within the normal and expected range for the time baby was in the womb.

Air leak. This refers to two different situations: (1) air leaking through damaged lung tissue into the chest cavity; or (2) air leaking during each ventilator breath around an endotracheal tube that is too small.

Anemia. The number of baby's red blood cells falls too low, making it harder for baby's bloodstream to deliver oxygen throughout the body. Anemia occurs in most preemies at some point during their stay in the NICU.

Apgar score. A score of 0 to 10 given to baby at the time of birth to assess how well baby initially transitioned to life outside the womb. Baby's heart rate, breathing, color, muscle tone, and reflexes are observed at one minute, five minutes, and sometimes ten minutes. A score of 7 to 10 means baby's heart, lungs, and other body systems kicked into gear right away. A score of 6 or less means that baby did not immediately transition well and was probably given resuscitative measures to get his heart, lungs, and circulation working.

Apnea. See As and Bs.

As and Bs. Apnea and bradycardia spells. A pause in infant's breathing that causes the heart rate to slow. These are common and easily treated.

Attending. An experienced physician in a teaching hospital who oversees the care in the NICU.

Bacteremia. An infection in the bloodstream.

BAER test. Brainstem auditory evoked response. A specialized hearing test.

Bagging or **bagged.** A mask is placed over baby's mouth, and an attached plastic "bag" is squeezed to pump breaths of air into baby's lungs. It may be done at the time of delivery to stimulate breathing (if baby doesn't begin breathing on her own) or if a problem occurs with baby's ventilator and a nurse needs to help the baby breathe while the ventilator machine is being adjusted.

Bililights or **biliblanket.** A row of lights or a blanket with light strips used to treat jaundice.

Bilirubin. A yellow pigment that builds up in baby's bloodstream as red blood cells are naturally broken down. It causes jaundice, or yellow color, to develop in baby's skin and eyes. Bilirubin levels are measured with a blood test.

Blood culture. A blood test to look for infection in the bloodstream.

Blood gas. A blood test to measure levels of oxygen and carbon dioxide. It is used to assess how well baby's lungs are working and to help coordinate the ventilator machine.

Blow-by. An oxygen tube pointed toward baby's mouth and nose to give baby a small amount of oxygen when needed.

BPD. Bronchopulmonary dysplasia. Lung disease or damage as a result of prematurity and ventilator therapy.

Bradycardia. Slowing of the heart rate, often triggered by an apnea (stop-breathing) episode.

Breast milk fortifier. Protein, vitamin, and mineral additive mixed with breast milk.

Bronchospasm. A tightening or spasm of the lung tubes (bronchi) that carry air deep into the lungs, causing wheezing and difficulty breathing. Treated with an inhaled bronchodilator medication.

Broviac catheter. A type of central line. See Central line.

Central line. An IV placed in the arm, groin, or chest that extends up into a large blood vessel. Different from a peripheral IV line, which goes only an inch or two into a small vein.

Cerebral palsy. Muscular and coordination problems as a result of brain injury.

Chest PT. Chest physiotherapy. Gentle clapping on the chest and back performed by a nurse or respiratory therapist to help baby cough up chest mucus.

Chest tube. A firm plastic tube inserted through a skin incision into the chest cavity. Used to drain out trapped blood or air that may be compressing the lungs.

CHF. Congestive heart failure. The heart is not functioning well enough to adequately pump blood and oxygen throughout the body.

CLD. Chronic lung disease. Term used in conjunction with BPD (bronchopulmonary dysplasia) to describe long-term lung disease. It is often due to prematurity and ventilator therapy.

CMV. (Cytomegalovirus). A virus that can cause birth defects or various medical problems for very premature babies. It can be passed from mother to baby during pregnancy. It is generally harmless to mild or moderately premature babies.

CNS. Central nervous system. Refers to the brain and spinal cord.

Colostomy. A surgical procedure that brings the end of the colon up and out to an opening in the skin of the abdomen. Stool comes out into a bag (instead of out of the anus into a diaper). This is necessary when part of the colon is severely damaged and needs to be surgically removed (usually as a result of NEC, a serious intestinal problem).

Colostrum. Protein- and antibody-rich fluid produced by the mom's breasts during the first few days after birth before regular breast milk comes in.

CPAP. Continuous positive airway pressure. Air is blown continuously through baby's nose or endotracheal tube to help keep baby's lungs open between breaths. Used in certain situations when baby doesn't need full ventilator support but can't breathe well enough on his own.

CSF. Cerebrospinal fluid. Fluid that circulates through the brain and spinal cord. It is often tested for infection with a spinal tap or lumbar puncture.

De-satting or **desaturation.** A drop in oxygen levels in baby's bloodstream. An alarm on baby's pulse ox monitor alerts the nurses if baby "de-sats."

Diuretic. Medication used to increase baby's urine production and help baby "pee off" excess body fluids.

Dopamine and **dobutamine.** Cardiac medications used to improve low blood pressure.

Echocardiogram or **Echo.** An ultrasound of the heart to assess heart function and look for heart defects. It is noninvasive

and painless, just like a prenatal ultrasound.

Edema. Swelling of any body part due to excess fluid collection. It may occur in the lungs, where it can be seen on a chest X-ray.

EEG. Electroencephalogram. Wires taped to baby's scalp measure the brain's electrical activity. It is used to assess brain function and evaluate seizures.

EKG. Electrocardiogram. Wires taped to baby's chest measure the electrical pattern of baby's heart beats.

Electrolytes. Various minerals that are crucial for overall body functions. They are measured in a blood test.

Epogen. A medication (erythropoetin) that stimulates red blood cell production. It is used to treat certain types of anemia.

ET tube. Endotracheal tube. A flexible plastic tube that is inserted through baby's nose or mouth and down into baby's lungs. The ET tube is hooked up to a ventilator machine.

Extubate. To remove the ET tube from baby. This procedure is usually done once baby shows she is ready to breathe on her own.

Feeder-growers. Stable preemies who no longer need any intensive care but continue to need assistance with learning to feed and other minor medical problems until they mature and reach a certain weight.

Feeding tube. A thin catheter inserted into baby's stomach through the mouth or nose to provide breast milk or formula.

Fellow. A doctor who is currently training to be a full neonatologist.

Flaring. Nasal flaring (widening of the nostrils with each breath), a sign that baby is having minor breathing difficulty.

Foley catheter. A flexible rubber tube inserted through the urethra (the opening where urine comes out) into the bladder and left in place to allow urine to drain.

Fontanel. The soft spot on top of baby's head.

Gavage feeding. Using a feeding tube (see above) to give baby breast milk or formula.

GI tract. Gastrointestinal tract. Refers to the stomach and intestines.

Group B strep. This bacteria lives in the vaginal area of some women and can be transmitted to a baby during delivery if the period of time since the mother's water broke is prolonged. Antibiotics given to a laboring woman are designed to prevent this. It is a very serious infection for a newborn.

G-tube. Gastrostomy tube. A large feeding tube that is surgically inserted through the abdominal wall into the stomach. It is used to provide gastrointestinal nutrition for infants who won't be able to feed by mouth for a long time.

Heart murmur. An extra humming sound heard while examining the heart. It is often a normal finding in preemies, but occasionally it can be a sign of a heart defect.

Heel stick. Pricking the heel to obtain several drops of blood for testing. It is an easier procedure than drawing blood from a vein with a needle.

Hematocrit. A blood test to check the number of red blood cells. It is used to test for anemia.

Hemoglobin. The part of the red blood cell that carries oxygen. It is measured with a blood test for anemia.

Hernia. Part of the intestines pushes against a weak part of the abdominal muscles and appears as a bulge underneath the skin around the belly button or in the groin. It is a common situation for preemies.

Human milk fortifier. Powder added to pumped breast milk containing extra protein, minerals, and vitamins.

Hydrocephalus. The buildup of fluid in the ventricles of the brain. It can cause neurologic problems if left untreated.

Hyperalimentation or **hyperal.** See TPN.

Hyperbilirubinemia. An abnormally high level of bilirubin in the bloodstream.

Hypoxia. A lack of oxygen, which can lead to brain damage.

Intracranial pressure. Pressure within the skull caused by buildup of fluid.

Intubate. To insert a breathing tube into baby's lungs.

Is and Os. The daily amount of fluids (IV and feeds) that baby takes in compared with how much baby pees and poops out.

IUGR. Intrauterine growth retardation. Term used to describe a baby who grows abnormally slowly in utero and is born smaller than expected.

IVH. Intraventricular hemorrhage. Bleeding within the ventricles (fluid spaces) in the brain.

Jaundice. Yellow skin and eyes caused by a buildup of bilirubin in the blood.

Kangaroo care. A method of caring for preemies that involves prolonged skin-to-skin contact.

Lanugo. Soft hair on the body of a preemie. It disappears as baby matures.

Lasix. A diuretic medication commonly used to increase urination in order to remove excess fluids from the body.

Leads. Monitor wires taped to baby's skin. You will often hear the nurse say that baby's monitor is alarming due to "loose leads."

LGA. Large for gestational age. A baby who is born weighing more than expected for her age in weeks.

LP. Lumbar puncture; another term for spinal tap. A needle is inserted between two vertebra in the lower back below the end of the spinal cord to collect spinal fluid for testing.

MCT oil. Medium-chain triglyceride oil. It can be added to breast milk or formula to provide extra calories for preemie growth.

Meningitis. An infection of the membrane surrounding the brain or spinal cord. It is diagnosed with a lumbar puncture, or spinal tap, to test the spinal fluid. It is treated with antibiotics.

Mucus plug. A thick plug of mucus that gets stuck within the lungs and blocks air flow.

Nasal canula. A plastic tube attached to two small nasal prongs that deliver oxygen to baby.

Nebulizer. A small machine used to give baby inhaled medications.

NEC. Necrotizing enterocolitis. A serious condition in which a portion of the intestines is damaged.

NG tube. Nasogastric tube. A thin rubber tube passed through baby's nose down into the stomach. It is used to feed baby breast milk or formula or to suction out excess stomach acid and mucus.

Nosocomial infection. An infection that is acquired from either a medical staff person or medical equipment in the hospital. Hand washing, gown wearing, and sterile procedures are designed to prevent nosocomial infections.

NPO. *Nil per os,* a Latin term meaning "nothing by mouth." It means a baby should not be given any feedings or liquids by mouth.

O2 sat. Oxygen saturation. The level of oxygen in baby's bloodstream. You will often hear the nurses say baby's "sats are stable."

Oxy-hood. A small plastic box or tent placed over baby's head. Oxygen is pumped into it to provide baby with extra oxygen.

PDA. Patent ductus arteriosus. A heart condition in which an extra fetal blood vessel next to the heart remains open instead of closing after birth as it should.

PEG tube. Percutaneous endoscopic gastrostomy tube. This tube is similar to a G-tube (see above), but it is inserted by a gastroenterologist in the NICU through a nonsurgical procedure.

Perc line. A percutaneous IV. See Central line.

Periodic breathing. A normal breathing pattern in preemies, consisting of rapid breaths followed by long pauses.

Peripheral IV. An IV in the arm, leg, or scalp that extends only 1 or 2 inches into the vein.

Periventricular leukomalacia. Damage to part of the brain caused by complications of prematurity.

Phototherapy. Light therapy for jaundice. See Bililights.

Platelets. A blood cell that creates blood clots and scabs to stop bleeding.

Pneumogram. A test while baby sleeps to assess problems with heart rate, breathing, and oxygen levels. It is used to evaluate apnea.

Pulmonary edema. A buildup of extra fluid in the lungs. It can be seen on a chest X-ray.

Pulse ox. Pulse oximeter. A monitor taped to baby's hand or foot that continuously measures oxygen levels.

RBCs. Red blood cells. Blood cells that carry oxygen. Levels are measured with a hemoglobin or hematocrit blood test.

RDS. Respiratory distress syndrome. Breathing trouble experienced by preemies whose lungs are immature.

Resident. A doctor who is training in general pediatrics or any other field but not specializing in neonatology.

Respirator. See Ventilator.

ROP. Retinopathy of prematurity. A weakening of the retina in young preemies. It can cause long-term problems with vision.

RSV. Respiratory syncytial virus. A virus that causes a severe chest cold and wheezing. It can be quite troublesome to a preemie with sensitive lungs.

Sepsis. A serious infection in the bloodstream that can affect various organs and cause complications. It is treated with antibiotics and intensive care.

SGA. Small for gestational age. A baby who is born weighing less than expected for his gestational age.

Short gut syndrome. Intestinal complications that require surgical removal of part of the intestines. The remaining intestines may not provide sufficient digestive function for baby as she grows.

Shunt or **VP shunt.** A thin tube, one end of which is surgically inserted through the skull into the ventricles (fluid collections within the brain), and the other end of which is maneuvered under the skin of the scalp, down the neck and chest, and eventually into the abdominal space, where it drains. It is used to continuously relieve the fluid buildup and pressure of hydrocephalus.

Sleep study. See Pneumogram.

Spinal tap. See LP.

Steroids. There are several common uses for steroids in the NICU. Their usefulness in decreasing inflammation throughout the body can be extremely beneficial for several preemie medical problems. Their benefits far outweigh any risks, and side effects are rare.

Strep, Group B. See Group B strep.

Surfactant. Substance produced in the lungs to assist with lung function. Often deficient in preemies, it can be given through an ET tube to help improve immature lungs.

Theophylline. A medication used to stimulate breathing in a preemie with apnea.

TPN. Total parenteral nutrition. Providing nutrition via a special intravenous fluid mix of carbohydrate, fat, protein, vitamins, and minerals. It is also known as hyperal.

Trachea. Windpipe. An ET tube used for mechanical ventilation extends down into the trachea.

Tube feeding. See Gavage feeding.

Umbilical catheter. An IV tube that is placed in the stump of the umbilical cord.

Urine dip. A dipstick test of baby's urine used to monitor baby's hydration status.

Ventilator or **vent.** A machine used to pump breaths of air through an ET tube into baby's lungs.

Ventricles. Refers to two different things: (1) the heart's two main chambers; or (2) the spaces in the brain that are filled with circulating fluid.

VP shunt. See Shunt.

WBCs. White blood cells. Blood cells that fight infection.

Resources

BABY CARRIERS

The Original BabySling
(800) 421-0526
www.AskDrSears.com. Visit our store.
www.nojo.com

BEDSIDE CO-SLEEPERS

Arm's Reach Co-Sleeper
(800) 954-9353 or (818) 879-9353
www.armsreach.com

BEDSIDE HAMMOCK

www.AmbyBaby.com

BREASTFEEDING

The Breastfeeding Book, by Martha Sears
and William Sears (Little, Brown, 2000)

La Leche League International (LLLI)
(800) 435-8316 or (847) 519-7730
www.lalecheleague.org

International Lactation Consultant Association (ILCA)
(919) 787-5181
www.ilca.org

Human Milk Bank Association of North
America
www.hmbana.org

CLOTHING AND ACCESSORIES FOR PREEMIES

www.earlybirds.com

www.preemie.com

www.snuggletown.com/preemie

www.tinybundles.com

GASTROESOPHAGEAL REFLUX (GERD)

Pediatric/Adolescent Gastroesophageal
Reflux Association (PAGER)
www.reflux.org

Reflux Wedges and Slings
www.tuckerdesigns.com

GRIEVING (RESOURCES FOR PARENTS WHO HAVE LOST A PREEMIE)

www.compassionatefriends.org

www.nationalshareoffice.com

PARENTING RESOURCES — GENERAL

The Baby Book: Everything You Need to Know About Your Baby from Birth to Age Two
By William, Martha, Robert, and James Sears
(Little, Brown, 2003)

www.AskDrSears.com

PREMATURE BABY — GENERAL RESOURCES

www.AskDrSears.com/preemie

www.preemie-L.com

RELAXATION MUSIC

Soothing Moments by Livesay, available at www.AskDrSears.com

RSV PROTECTION

www.rsvprotection.com

TWINS AND MULTIPLES

M.O.S.T. (Mothers of Supertwins)
A national nonprofit organization providing information, resources, empathy, and support to families with triplets or more.
www.MOSTonline.org.

National Organization of Mothers of Twins Clubs
(877) 540-2200 or (615) 595-0936
www.nomotc.org

Index

William Sears, M.D., received his pediatric training at Harvard Medical School's Children's Hospital and Toronto's Hospital for Sick Children, where he was Associate Ward Chief of the Newborn Intensive Care Unit. He has practiced as a pediatrician for more than thirty years. Martha Sears is a registered nurse, childbirth educator, and breastfeeding consultant. The Searses are the parents of eight children and coauthors of thirty-two books. Their sons Dr. Robert Sears, father of three, and Dr. James Sears, father of two, are both board-certified pediatricians at the Sears Family Pediatric Practice in San Clemente, California, and coauthors of *The Baby Book*. All four authors live in Southern California.